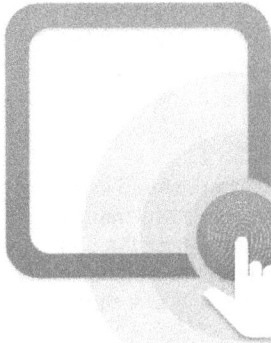 **TOUCH**

TO KNOW

https://TouchToKnow.io

First published by Busybird Publishing 2019
Copyright © 2019 Len Kennedy

ISBN
Hardback: 978-1-925949-55-1
Paperback: 978-1-925949-90-2
Ebook: 978-1-925949-23-0

Cover image: Kev Howlett
Cover design: Busybird Publishing
Layout and typesetting: Busybird Publishing

Busybird Publishing
2/118 Para Road
Montmorency, Victoria
Australia 3094
www.busybird.com.au

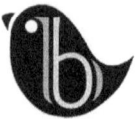

Hidden HOSPITAL HAZARDS

Saving Lives and Improving Margins

Len Kennedy
Founder & CEO of Touch to Know

This book is dedicated to reducing avoidable errors in hospitals.

Contents

Foreword

To the reader,

Over a long and distinguished career in the health industry, Len Kennedy has constantly challenged and prodded 'the system' to make it better.

Len is an insightful man, a fact that will become clear, as you read this book.

You will see his ability to tackle a problem from all sides using a breadth of knowledge drawn from his extensive academic study and industry experience.

In this book, Len clearly articulates issues facing the health industry and takes you on a problem-solving journey that you will find both logical and beautifully simple.

I commend this book to you.

Geoff Fazakerley
Executive Director Diagnostic Services and Infrastructure, Cabrini Health Care.

With the increasing "consumerization" of healthcare – consumers demanding the same level of experience from the industry as they get elsewhere in the economy – it's time for hospitals to embrace what Len Kennedy calls "touch-to-know" technology.

The state-of-the-art in today's Experience Economy requires digitizing information, processes, and offerings to bring both efficiencies to companies and more customized offerings to individuals.

It is time for hospitals to embrace this touch-to-know world to free up personnel – clinical and non-clinical – to do what they are called to do: care for patients.

– B. Joseph Pine II
co-author of
The Experience Economy and Infinite Possibility: Creating Customer Value on the Digital Frontier

Introduction

We Live in a
'Touch-to-Know' World

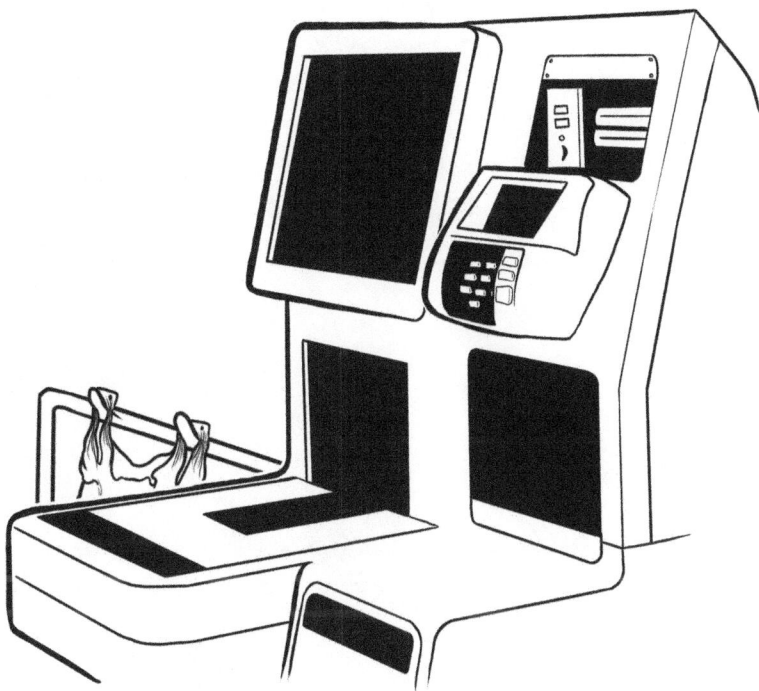

Whether you're shopping for corn flakes, looking for the nearest petrol station, or the best route to take for a meeting, you probably touch your phone before you act on your impulse. Touch-to-know capability has become a way of life.

I have used the term 'touch-to-know' to highlight how smartphones have reshaped many aspects of our lives.

Our smartphones have eliminated many of the manual processes previously used for hailing a ride, ordering food or clothing or just about anything else online and to perform many daily tasks.

The innovative use of smartphones has removed inconveniences like queuing at check-out counters, dealing with cash transactions, dealing with paperwork or any hurdles to get information. It has made searching as easy as touching our phones. We do all of this by keying the barest information ourselves. Instead, information is gathered from the context in which we do things.

We have adopted smartphones willingly and seamlessly. Such adoption requires no training, education program, enforcement of rules and regulations or other change management programs. In fact, my first recollection of the introduction of mobile phones was their prohibition in many places, especially in hospitals.

I have worked in Australian hospitals for three decades as a supply chain professional and business process expert, implementing new technology to improve hospital efficiency and compliance. Yet, no implementation was ever adopted as seamlessly and as willingly as we adopted smartphones. In hospitals, in order to improve efficiency and compliance, we use extensive change management initiatives, education programs, and enlist program champions. We resort to written rules, regulations, and often even legislation.

As systems experts, we tend to think in terms of business margins. Generally speaking, we see value in the visible contribution that's made between the cost of delivering a service and the price charged for providing it. However, there are other valuable contributions as well. If we're not cognisant of the finer contributions of the work being done, we unknowingly placed hidden hazards in the way of everyone – patients, visitors and clinicians.

For instance, before the introduction of smartphones, we were unaware of the time we lost between meetings. With our ability to schedule meetings more conveniently and appropriately on our smartphones, such gaps proved to be extremely valuable to us. I have called the uncovering of these gaps 'touch-to-know' capability.

'Touch-to-know' capability has not made any inroads into hospital life in situations where they could impact, such as:

- Finding the way from the hospital car park to a physician's office

- Finding the bedside of a friend who's been admitted for a procedure

- Filling out forms before being admitted to the hospital or even to see a physician

- Finding equipment or medical items that have already been received in the hospital, but cannot be tracked or traced for patient care

Hospitals are making a push to address these inconveniences by implementing electronic medical records. Yet, the focus on how we implement things still has not changed. Hospital, administrators have pushed the administrative burden onto clinicians. This is a steep hill to climb because inputting information into computers takes nurses and clinicians twice as long as using paper forms. Designers force clinicians to follow computer processes designed to prevent errors in collecting information that may be useful at some point in the process.

David Price, an author and advocate for using new technologies describes his physician's frustrations with such processes in a Trust Hospital in the UK.[1]

'I previously visited my doctor to ask for some blood tests since I was struggling to shake off a virus. In order to simply attach a label to my blood going off to the test lab, she had to follow a screen-by-screen set of questions: Had I been abroad recently? (If yes to "the Far East", test for avian flu). Had I had any unusual bowel motions? (If yes, test for coeliac disease). It was fairly comical to see her trying to request a test for *Clostridium difficile*, only to be told that the computer said "no".'

As the lab labels spewed out of her printer, she was instructed to 'affix label A to red vial', and so on… okay, we know that mistakes happen, but seeing 7 years of training and 20-years'professional practice reduced to a series of tick boxes must be quite dispiriting.

From this snippet, it becomes clear that there is a disparity about the relevance of the information to the end-user and the designer of the system. Designers collect information just in case it may be useful at some point, whereas end-users need information only to perform the work at hand. This is the central issue that this book addresses – 'How to collect information for better treatment without hindering performance?'

The Content of This Book

This book takes you on a problem-solving journey that is informed by practical experience gained from dealing with patients, their relatives, nurses, clinical specialists, physicians and hospital administrators.

In Chapter 1, this book begins with my surprise finding that I ought to have put end-user's needs, their capabilities, and behaviours first, and then designed work flows to accommodate those needs, capabilities and ways of behaving.

With that insight gained, Chapter 2 deals with the ways in which technology and digitising information about materials could address the challenges faced by hospital administrators and end-users.

Chapter 3 looks at what hospitals are currently doing and suggests what they ought to do instead.

Chapter 4 suggests how peripheral databases help to minimise data entry for end-users. The chapter shows how information can influence our thinking and behaviours.

Chapter 5 explores how we can use technology to simplify patient safety, influence safe behaviour, and share information with working peers for safety.

Chapter 6 focuses on the use of context-aware apps to prompt carers for task completion when they're interrupted by other emergencies. These apps expose hidden hazards that may be encountered at the patient's bedside.

Chapter 7 shows how hospital challenges can be overcome by adopting suitable technology that automates information collection without getting in the way of the work being performed.

Chapter 8 summarises how ten hidden hospital hazards can be suitably addressed with the adoption of context-aware computers and sensors.

In the conclusion, we look at Charles Conn and Robert McLean's seven step process to iterate, prioritise and solve many of the unresolved problems that hospitals still face.[2] We will use this iterative model in the next two books of the series to address other hospital challenges. In book two of this series, we will delve deeper into procedure costing and inventory management accuracy. In book three of the series, we will delve into a different business model that hospitals can use to improve their margins and yet provide their patients and physicians with the widest choice of materials and services they need, and at lower costs.

1

A Fundamental Surprise

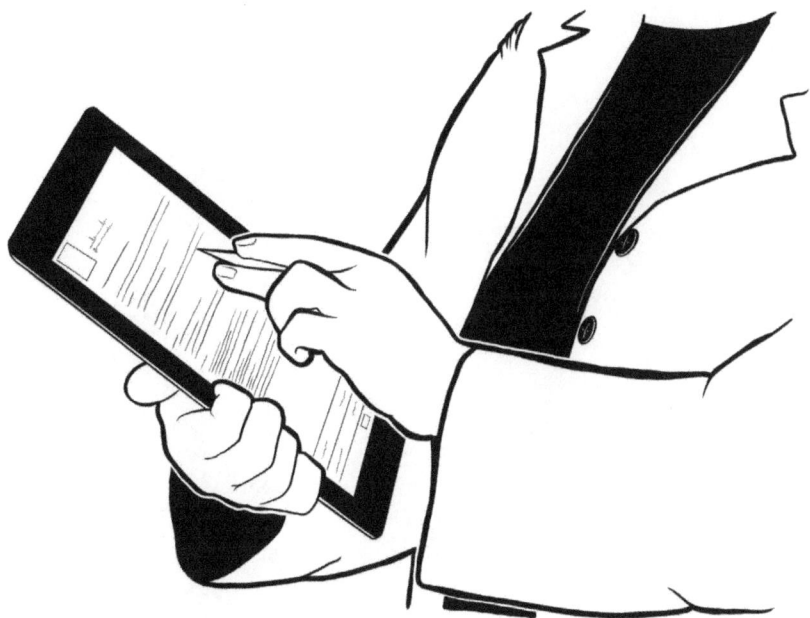

In my introduction, I pointed out that touch-to-know capability has not yet reached hospitals. I observed that this was strange when technology is changing behaviour in completely new ways, even to the point where campaigns and legislation fail consistently.[3] Yet hospital executives are not convinced that technology can change behaviour, increase patient safety, and improve hospital margins more easily than mandates can.[4] Technology in hospitals is often used to force behaviour change. Forcing change in this way often creates resistance and pushback in the form of workarounds.[5] (Something which I've been guilty of.)

Workarounds

Workarounds are often considered a necessary part of work since they appear to smooth workflow hindrances and get the job done. Yet, they can be potentially harmful. Nurses, in particular, obtain a great deal of professional satisfaction from fixing system problems, often using workarounds. These problems include missing or broken equipment, missing or incomplete supplies, missing or incorrect information, waiting for people or equipment to arrive, and other multiple demands on their time. Unfortunately, these workarounds can carry severe penalties.

James Reason, an international expert on safety, in his book on the human contribution to errors reported that behaviour researchers, Tucker and Edmondson observed the work of 26 nurses in nine hospitals to investigate how nurses dealt with problems that impeded patient care. In 93% of observed instances, nurses found short-term local fixes that enabled them to continue caring for their patients, but which did not tackle the underlying organisational shortcomings. Another strategy used on 42% of occasions was to seek assistance from another nurse rather than a more senior person who could do something about the root problem. In both cases, an opportunity for improving the system was lost and errors accumulated as a result.[6]

The Accumulation of Error

James Reason found from many case studies he and colleagues had studied that major disasters are rarely caused by any one factor. Disasters are caused from the combination of various diverse events that come together locally. Although each single factor is insufficient in itself, it is the accumulative effect that can be crippling.[7]

Reason sees similarities between hospital decision-making and the lifestyle choices we make. In both cases, it's the accumulation of small mistakes that eventually wreaks havoc. Adverse events and diseases arise from the combination of various diverse events that come together locally.[8]

In hospitals, computers were introduced as a tool to assist clinicians to perform their tasks more easily. But because computers need busy clinicians to input constantly changing information into them, computers actually distract clinicians from their primary task of patient care, and this encourage workarounds. Some practitioners claim that the need to input information into computers has doubled the workload of clinicians.[9]

Active and Latent Errors

James Reason makes an important distinction between active errors and latent errors. This distinction can help prevent errors at the point of insertion into a system. Active errors are usually associated with the performance of people at the frontline; in hospitals, these would be the clinicians and nurses dealing with the patient. Their actions have an immediate impact on the system. Latent errors are generated by people that are far removed from the patient. These would be the high level decision-makers and architects of systems and processes. Such errors lie dormant for a long time, only making their presence felt when they combine with active errors at the local level to trigger an accident.

Financial Difficulty

I'd been working in hospitals as a supply chain professional for approximately three decades when the hospital financial situation had deteriorated sufficiently for me to venture outside my immediate area of concern – which was the supply of medical consumables. I now felt that I had to see how these items were being used. In my then role all I saw was the financial impact of my purchases. As Dave Gray, the author and management consultant says, 'looking at a result tells us very little about the causes that lead to that result.' What really matters are the activities that generate the profit or the activities that destroy value.[10]

Anecdotally, I and other hospital supply chain professionals, believed that a major contributor to our financial predicament was inaccurate procedure costing. No hospital, due to the volume of transactions, could easily identify the cost of each individual procedure.[11] The 'workaround' was to aggregate the cost of supplies. But aggregation did not give us, as procurement specialists, a handle to correct material costs. To negotiate prices with vendors, we needed granular costing and a guarantee that we would actually use the product. At present, most hospital executives cannot provide this.

Human Error

At no time in those 30 years as a supply chain professional did I think asking nurses to list the items they used could contribute to human error in the operating suites. I felt that asking nurses to input information into computers was a reasonable demand. To make this task easier, I thought, like in supermarkets, nurses could use touchscreens and barcode scanning to list the items they used. I felt I was uniquely qualified to provide such a system.

In 1999, I had, as part of a three person team, set up an enterprise resource planning (ERP) system to manage financials, warehousing and distribution of materials in the hospital. Between 2000 and 2003, I installed Pyxis, the largest automated dispensing system for pharmaceutical drugs and high-value medical consumables in South-East Asia at the time. Intermittently, over a 10-year-period, I also developed and implemented several other software solutions to automate various aspects of the hospital supply chain.

Pre-preparation

In April 2011, six months before a visit to the operating suites, I began to create a database that I called MediDataCapture. I visualised this database as an integration engine that would combine information from the various hospital systems to eventually produce procedure costing documents. Operating suites receive materials from different routes and information from various systems. For instance, there's the loan kit management system, the procedure card system, the case cart system, the sterilising system, the patient management system, the theatre booking system, and the ERP system that manages financials, materials inventory, and materials distribution and reordering. MediDataCapture was to provide the frontend interface for the touchscreens and barcode scanning in the operating suite.

I didn't realise that I was setting myself up for a fundamental surprise.

A Significant Learning Experience

Israeli social scientist, Zvi Lanir coined the term 'fundamental surprise' to describe a situation that causes us to reappraise our perception of the world and our reality.[12]

To test my ideas about MediDataCapture, I was given permission to demonstrate how easy it was to list the items used in a procedure so the information could then be used for clinical, financial and supply chain decision-making.

I had come to the operation suite fully prepared for the task at hand. I had the latest touchscreen tablet, preloaded with all the information for materials that could possibly be used for the procedure. At the backend, MediDataCapture would consolidate information from other systems to produce a consolidated procedure costing document in real time, giving us immediate feedback.

The procedure in this instance was for a hip-replacement for a 62-year-old man, Sam (not his real name). Before the procedure began, the surgeon held Sam's hand and explained what he and his team would do, explained my role and got Sam's consent for me to be present. He assured Sam that he was in safe, capable hands. The surgeon said that with the anaesthesia, he would not feel any pain or have any consciousness of the procedure.

When the procedure began, Sam was intubated, which involves inserting a tube down the trachea to prevent involuntary suffocation. Sam suffered a heart attack. The resuscitation team brought Sam back to life and the procedure continued.

Two incidents during the procedure caused me some concern. The surgeon was handed a defective scope, meaning another had to be found. Then, when the surgeon wanted to set the new hip in place, two screws, previously checked and validated as being on the operating tray, were missing. Instead, we had two screws of the wrong size.

Fortunately, the correct screws were located and the procedure completed. On the surface, all had gone well; however, had these two errors not been corrected, the patient would have suffered. The procedure would have had to be stopped and then recommenced another day.

A few days later, I saw Sam walking effortlessly down the hospital corridors.

Cause for Concern

Most errors that take place in patient care cause no harm. However, if small errors (like the above example) are not taken as seriously as severe errors, this could lull us into a sense of complacency. When any error takes place it must alert us to the possibility that a serious event could have occurred. The more I have reflected on this, the more I realised that unnecessary demands on clinicians to collect information at the point of care was a cause for concern.[13]

A Mental Slip

The procedure I witnessed had taken a little over one hour and forty-five minutes. I returned to my office to analyse the procedure costs. All I had listed was the patient's unique reference number and the type of procedure. I had no other details other than the feeds from the systems that were interfaced with MediDataCapture. To my surprise, I had not listed a single item used during the procedure. Without listing the items used, my efforts were useless.

I had suffered what James Reason and Don Norman call a mental slip.[14] I now realised, as Kevin Ashton had discovered decades earlier, that people who focused on other tasks do not have time to update computers with constantly changing data. [15] I like the nurses and clinicians was concerned only with the patient's wellbeing, everything else was of no concern.

It's not as though nurses hadn't repeatedly pointed this out. But I had, like so many others in hospitals, been protected by a psychological and physical distance[16] from the task, fallen foul of the 'fundamental attribution error'[17] of blaming nurses for not doing things that they were not humanly capable of consistently doing.[18]

Fundamental Attribution Error

What I learnt from visiting the operation suite was that we tend to judge ourselves by our intentions, but judge others by their actions. Because nurses did not accurately list the items they used during a procedure, I had misread their intentions. Don Norman, who is best known as an expert in the field of design, useability engineering, and cognitive science, believes that when we encounter a problem with physical objects, we tend to look for root causes and eliminate them. But where people are concerned, we design work in unnatural ways, blame them when they fail, and then continue doing things as we've always done.[19]

Knowing by Doing

I now realised the difference between 'knowing' and 'knowing from experience'. Prior to this, I had known of nurses complaining about lack of time but I hadn't experienced for myself what they were complaining about. Having visited our operating suites and experienced for myself the difficulty of performing a task when focusing on the patient on the table, I knew how impractical it was to list used items during the procedure.

Prior to visiting the operation suite, I hadn't realised how difficult it was to multi-task in that environment. I could now see that focusing on the patient made it difficult to consistently perform other unrelated tasks. In 1999, when I had first implemented JD Edwards, the hospital enterprise resource planning software, I couldn't understand why nurses constantly asked, 'Why must we work for JD Edwards, why can't JDE work for us?' Now given my experience, I did.

I was now on a quest of a different kind. I asked myself, 'How could I, without distracting nurses and clinicians from caring for patients, get a list of materials used during a procedure?' What other benefits could such a system provide? How could MediDataCapture become context-aware?

Context-Aware Computers

I came across context-aware computers in two different industries. These computers used sensors to read information broadcast by ultra-high frequency radio identification (UHF-RFID) tags attached to the physical product. The information from the tags was made available to different parts of the organisation by using the internet.

When the Qantas Q Bag Tags were introduced, you no longer needed to attach a temporary baggage tag to your bags each time you flew. You could just drop your bags at the bag drop and go. The tag synchronised your details with your boarding pass and your baggage.

Libraries use passive ultra-high frequency radio frequency tags (UHF-RFID) attached to the spines of their books. The unique identification number on each chip is matched with the borrower's details and automatically checks-in the books when dropped into the chutes. No human intervention other than the chute-drop is needed.

The MediDataCapture Pilot

In April 2012, MediDataCapture, similar to library systems, was interfaced with a cloud-based UHF-RFID system that tracked tags as they moved through the hospital.

Because materials vendors did not tag their product, I implemented a process for all items received at the hospital to be individually RFID tagged by a storeperson. The UHF-RFID tags were attached to the sterile packaging of each tagged item. When the item was used and the packaging was discarded, sensors in the trash area of the hospital automatically created a list of items discarded. The information was fed back to MediDataCapture and to JD Edwards, the hospital enterprise resource planning system, for replenishing the used items.

In the first year, the MediDataCapture pilot saved the hospital $1.3 million. These savings were achieved in ways as described here.

- Storage costs were reduced by $700,000 because expensive automated dispensing units that housed medical consumables were no longer required to track and trace items.

- In Australia, hospitals are reimbursed the cost of prosthetics used in a procedure. Because the prosthetic items are not always listed, claims leakage to the extent of $583,000 was prevented.

- There was improvement in the ability to track and trace items (valued at $144,000) so that they could be returned to manufacturers before their use-by dates.

- Finally, due to picking efficiency, overtime in the supply department was reduced by $120,000. Further savings in other areas of the hospital were not quantified.

For the purpose of this book, I define digitisation as the representation of physical objects, information, and media as computer data.

I realised that by making information about materials used in the hospital available electronically, the hospital could solve previously difficult problems related to materials and patient care.

By using such digitised material information with context-aware computers, we could improve patient safety, reduce human error, change behaviour, and transform the hospital business model.

Further on, we will explore how UHF-RFID can be used as the infrastructure to enhance patient safety and bring touch-to-know capability to a hospital.

Solving Simple Problems

Although healthcare is awash with technology, Clayton Christensen and his colleagues have found that successful adoption occurs only when the simple problems are solved first.[20]

With this in mind, listing materials used in a procedure serves as the basis for incremental adoption of a simple problem that can lead to solving more and more complex problems in the hospital environment.

Christensen identifies a consistent pattern for adoption in all industries and this is consistent for healthcare as well. Transformation is brought about by three elements, as seen in the figure on the next page.

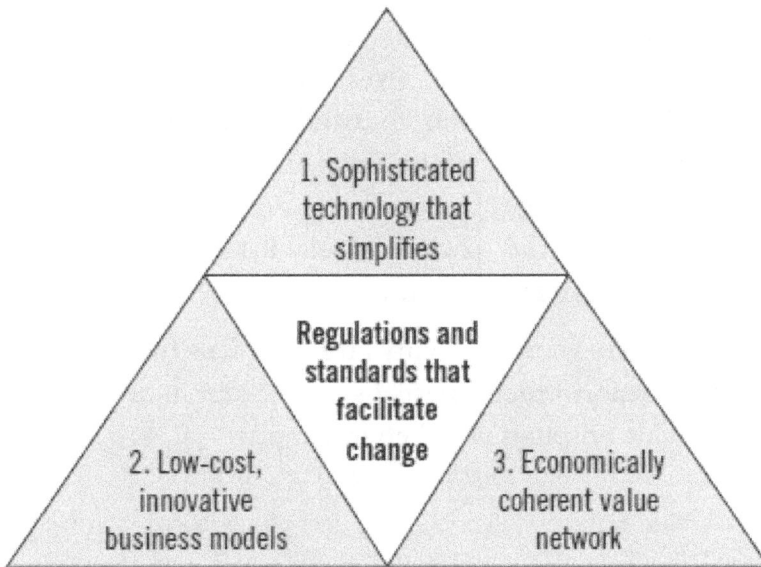

Elements for adoption

Sophisticated technology simplifies and makes routine the solutions to problems that were previously difficult to contend with.

Such simplification leads to the adoption of new business models that provides these products and services in more affordable and conveniently accessible formats using value networks. In this way, technology becomes a ubiquitous part of our personal lives and in the work life of hospitals.

Summary

- Hospitals need context-aware computers that harvest data from the natural flow of work without distracting clinicians and nurses from their primary task of patient care. This is possible if hospitals digitise the information of all the materials that they use.

- Context-aware computers can provide touch-to-know capability that gives clinicians immediate feedback and prompts to avoid human error, and improve patient safety. Immediate feedback on poor work design reduces 'latent errors'[21] that occur because of the psychological distance between decision-making and patient care.

- Touch-to-know capability gives hospitals the ability to transform their internal supply chain in order to provide hospitals with better margins.

2

Technology That Simplifies

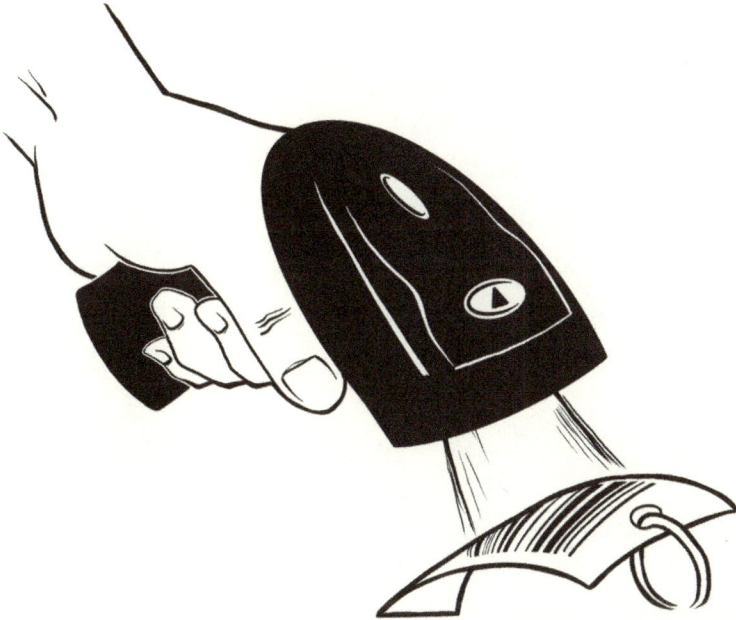

In this chapter, I will expand on why technology that simplifies internal supply chain functions is important for hospitals and why digitisation of materials using UHF-RFID is the first step that must be taken to benefit from the Internet of Things (IoT).

Automated Data Entry

Most people think of the Internet of Things as a large set of connected devices. This belies the more important aspect of IoT. The Internet of Things is a ubiquitous sensor network that supplements human data entry via keyboards and other interfaces with automatic data capture. Because RFID works silently in the background, most of us are not aware of its existence.[22]

Benedict Evans, consultant and long-time mobile analyst and pundit who works with Andreessen Horowitz, identified that most adults possesses a smartphone.[23] Enu Waktola – who works with RAIN-RFID, a global alliance promoting the universal adoption of UHF-RFID technology – points out in contrast, that there are about a billion more RFID tags sold each year than mobile phones and yet nobody even notices this important point.[24]

The Internet of Things (IoT)

Calum McClelland, editor of *IoT For All* and the business director of Leverage says, 'An internet connection is a wonderful thing, it gives us all sorts of benefits that just weren't possible before. If you're old enough, think of your cell phone before it was a smartphone. You could call and you could text, sure, but you couldn't read any book, watch any movie, or listen to any song, all in the palm of your hand. And that's just to name a few of the incredible things your smartphone can do. The point is that connecting something to the internet yields many amazing benefits. We've all seen these benefits with our smartphones, laptops, and tablets, but this is true for everything else too.'[25]

These are of course examples from our personal lives as consumers; however, the McKinsey Global Institute says business applications of IoT have greater economic potential than consumer applications.[26] But with businesses, it appears to be a case of 'out of sight, out of mind'.

Out of Sight, Out of Mind

Enu Waktola interviewed Kevin Ashton to find out why, when RFID has connected more than 15 billion things, people outside the RFID industry do not equate RFID with the Internet of Things.[27]

Ashton said it was hard to recall how the world had changed since 1999 when he was trying to build the Internet of Things. When Ashton first started working on IoT, internet access was mainly dial-up. Cellular networks were for voice and SMS, there was no wi-fi, and there was little or no digital photography, GPS was only for military use at the time. There weren't even any DVDs. To watch a movie at home you had to go to Blockbuster and hope you'd find the video-cassette you wanted to rent.

Now we take high-bandwidth wireless networking, digital media, and sensors like digital cameras and GPS for granted. With all this, RFID has progressed too. What was once expensive can be purchased cheaply. This fact does not appear to have dawned on the majority of hospital executives.

Christensen suggests that a good way understand the relevance of such progress is to deconstruct the organisation's mission by asking, 'What are the specific jobs to be done?' By clearly defining jobs, people will autonomously do what they need to do.[28]

In this regard, 'jobs to be done' must satisfy five specific criteria in a hospital:

Jobs to be Done

1. The job must assist a nurse or clinician in progressing towards an end result in a given set of circumstances.

2. For the innovation to be successful, it must enable the nurse's desired progress, resolve their struggle, and fulfil unmet aspirations. The solution must fulfil formerly inadequate or non-existent solutions.

3. These jobs, in addition to the functional needs, must satisfy social and emotional dimensions. These may be even more powerful than the functional need.

4. Because these jobs occur in the daily flow of work, the context is central and becomes the unit of innovation at work. It is not a customer characteristic, product attribute, new technology or trend.

5. The job to be done must not be a discrete event, it must be ongoing and recurring.

I have listed ten of these jobs to be done, as unresolved challenges that I consider must be resolved in hospitals.

1 – Reduce Materials Costs

Currently hospitals cannot, as I pointed out in my introduction, cost individual procedures, nor can they accurately account for inventory.[29] Instead, as a workaround, hospital costs are aggregated. Aggregating costs only enables hospitals to manage their cashflow but not to take corrective action at the individual procedure level. Hence, hospitals are unable to identify or explain why costs vary from procedure to procedure, or even for the same procedure, and cannot take corrective action to reduce costs.[30] Hospital workarounds[31] carry heavy hidden penalties[32], which we will explore throughout the course of this book.

No organisation can survive in the long term without an accurate means of costing their services. The gap between what ought to be done and what is actually done is exemplified by poor hospital margins.[33]

2 – Hiding Inventory

Hospitals use thousands of items for patient care. These items are normally stored in treatment rooms. However, the items do not remain on the shelves for long since nurses need unrestricted access to materials to provide good care.

It is humanly impossible to track items once they leave the treatment room because they are in constant circulation. As a result, nurses take defensive action by hiding inventory.[34] This creates a million-dollar black hole in hospital budgets.[35] There is other flow on effects as well:

- One-third of all hospital procedures get postponed or cancelled.
- Nurses spend one-fifth of their working days looking for items.

- Sixty percent of all moveable assets and medical items are hidden, resulting in unnecessary purchases of items that hospitals already possess and eventual obsolescence.

- There is negative impact on patient care.

3 – No Time, No Space, No Materials

If hospitals digitise their supply chains (that is, digitising information about materials), they'll be able to convert their current limitations, the experience of having 'no-time, no-space and no-materials', into assets.[36] They will be able to apply a similar business model that many new-age businesses are successfully using. New-age businesses are businesses that own limited assets as compared to other businesses that have invested in heavy assets in order to manufacture products or provide services.

Airbnb and Uber have shown us that access to other peoples' assets (with permission) is more important than owning the assets. Their business model helps people utilise their time, space and materials more appropriately.[37] Hospitals could quite easily do the same with a small investment in technology or by partnering with a third party logistics provider for a wider impact beyond a single hospital to several similarly networked hospitals served by the same provider to gain the exponential benefits of network effects.[38]

4 – Keeping Patients Safe

Patient safety is a major concern for hospital administrators. Hospitals must find ways and means to improve safety.[39] Many hospitals are going down the digital pathway by using electronic medical records.[40] This approach has had mixed results because clinicians still have to input large amounts of constantly changing information using manual interventions such as barcode scanning.

Using computers as brains without sensors to automatically capture information from the world around us is still 20th-century thinking.[41] This book argues that when materials are digitised and computers are linked to the internet through sensors, manual data entry will be eliminated. Such digitisation will vastly improve accuracy and will pay tremendous dividends both in terms of safety and financial benefits.

5 – Avoiding Human Error

In 2000, the Institute of Medicine released a report, 'To Err is Human', which asserted that the problem of medical errors is not that bad people are in healthcare, it's that good people are working in bad systems that need to be made safer.[42] Yet hospitals lack sufficient technological support systems to help avoid such accidents.

Today, accident prevention has become more possible because computers can be provided with sensors to make sense of the environment around them. When connected to the internet, information can be consolidated to amplify both local knowledge and application software knowledge to enable clinicians to work safely in spite of the many distractions in their work environment.[43]

6 – Reducing Feedback Delay

We have come to accept the influence computers and software can have on our behaviour and thinking. B J Fogg (a behaviour scientist) first introduced this concept in the 90s.[44] His thinking has morphed into behaviour design, which comprises of a set of models for understanding how human behaviour works. His methods are being used by innovators to create many useful products to help us overcome barriers so successful behavioural change can take place.[45]

This is particularly important in situations where active and passive errors can lie dormant within a system for a long time. Harm only occurs when the accumulation of failures to correct these errors combine with other factors to cause an unforeseen event.[46] In such circumstances, it is important to neutralise each error as they occur.[47]

The common thread that runs through such events is feedback delay between behaviour and outcomes. James Clear calls this 'the plateau of latent potential'.[48] It occurs when we cannot see the tangible outcomes of deviations immediately and then these deviations become the norm.

7 – Avoiding Hospital Workarounds

Behaviour design is particularly relevant to hospital workarounds. Nurses regularly encounter many small problems which, if not attended to immediately, could cripple the functioning of a hospital. The workarounds the nurses employ appear to iron out the wrinkles in systems and smooth services, but in reality, it's the small problems that nurses work around that eventually damage the hospital.[49]

Small problems often don't seem important enough to warrant attention. But because they don't get addressed, they must be worked around. These workarounds consume at least 20% of an employee's day[50] and carry safety, financial, and process penalties, as I have already pointed out.

8 – Physician Preference Items

All hospitals face tensions between the need to grant clinicians the widest possible choice of items to use for patient care, and the need to restrict choice through standardisation. The main driver for this tension is the cost of goods.

Clinicians prefer items that usually have a higher cost. Procurement officers believe that by standardising items, they get preferential pricing for volume. Suppliers offer hospitals preferential pricing that is subject to commercial-in-confidence agreements. Paradoxically, because vendors make it difficult to compare product equivalence, claiming product differentiation, hospitals are often forced to buy items that are not preferentially priced because vendors not on the approved list claim that their product must be purchased as their items are better for patient care.[51]

With digitisation process, it will become possible to share the cost per procedure data and success outcomes with physicians that use different items and different processes. Such peer reviews will eventually remove the tensions between the widest choice of product and standardisation. This echoes the sentiments of Jeff Bezos (CEO of Amazon): '[Hospitals] make money when [they] help customers make purchase decisions.' This sentiment has made Amazon the most successful online company in the world.[52]

9 – Siloed Information

Because different departments have their own pool of information about products, communication between the operating suites, sterilising department and materials management is seen as problematic.[53]

Most IT processes affect data quality negatively. Data quality continuously deteriorates unless there's an ongoing systematic program to monitor it and prevent deterioration.[54] Digitising materials and storing this information in the cloud this will provide all departments with a single source of synchronised data for effective communication and to track and trace items in real time.

To track an item is to define its current location and to trace an item is to be able to identify where it has been at different points of time.[55] Both aspects of this information are important for item useability, patient safety and efficient process flow.

10 – Improving Hospital Margins

Hospitals are in serious financial trouble.[56] If they want to maintain affordability, they must find ways to reduce costs and improve their margins. They can do this by looking inwards at their current processes to find ways to eliminate duplication of effort. They can also look outwards to see what other businesses are doing to improve their margins.

Research shows that most hospitals are already looking inwards to improve supply chains. This is a good starting place because material costs, as pointed out already, are the second largest area of expenditure in hospitals.[57]

I believe that hospitals should not only look inward, but outwards, particularly at marketplace platforms, the new-age business models.

These new-age business models would allow hospitals to capitalise on network effects and improve margins by using others' assets like Airbnb and Uber do.

Hospitals must strive to divest themselves of all assets except a few core ones essential to their business. This is similar to the approach taken by new-age businesses like Google, Apple, Facebook and Amazon.[58] These aspects of digitisation, not fully dealt with in this particular book, will be dealt with later in this series.

Digital Technology

Digital technology, as Joseph Pine and Kim Korn say, differs from other technology due to the following distinctive characteristics:[59]

1. **Bits are immaterial.** They weigh nothing, and cost little to store and replicate.

2. **Bits are easily integrated.** Any digital device can communicate with another, almost instantaneously following standard protocols. For instance, our smartphone can now be used to control appliances in our homes, such as lighting and air-conditioning. If we're on the road, GPS and location services assist us to find our way and reroute the journey with prompts if we take a wrong turn. I've referred to this as touch-to-know capability, but apps now even allow verbal requests if touch is inconvenient.

3. **Bits are cheap when it comes to imagining, experimentation, and prototyping.** Those of us who have used the old typewriters will recall how difficult it was to correct typing errors. Now with the digital capability of computers, we can play around with documents without even incurring the cost of printing. Even with physical goods, we can design, prototype, and test without incurring the cost of physical production until we're ready.

4. **Bits are easily modified, combined, improved and customised.** Notice how easily our computers and devices are upgraded with the latest software and digital tools we use.

5. **Bits are abundant.** Once we produce something digitally, we can, in effect, have an infinite supply. There is no physical limit to the number of copies we can produce and send out and share. Compare this with physical goods, their production, storage, and logistics costs.

Zeroes and ones talk to zeroes and ones. While this provides a common language for different systems to talk and communicate with each other, in reality this must be orchestrated using internet and transfer protocols.

Orchestration

Kevin Ashton, after helping Procter and Gamble – a multinational fast-moving consumer goods company – successfully restock shelves devoted his time to building the Internet of Things.[60] Ashton says, 'Building the Internet of Things was slow and hard, fraught with politics, infested with mistakes, unconnected to grand plans or strategies. I learned to succeed by learning to fail. I learnt to expect conflict. I learned not to be surprised by adversity but to prepare for it.'

Similarly, digitising the hospital supply chain will face adversity from many quarters within the organisation if not orchestrated carefully.

Poor ERP Stories

I suspect that orchestration for hospitals is difficult because hospital executives have long memories and are still conflicted by the memory of poor computer system integrations of the past. Horror stories abound[61] and we experience difficulty with these systems even today. In Australia, as recently as 2017–18, a large medical vendor and a third party logistics warehousing and distribution company could not synchronise their information to ship the product to hospitals. The problems took in excess of a year to fix, and the vendor lost substantial business, causing it to also lose its status as a preferred vendor.

I suspect resistance can be overcome by progressively tackling unresolved hospital challenges. These are jobs that all of us could rally around.

The Approach to Adoption

Gerardo Aue, Stefan Biesdorf, and Nicolaus Henke, from McKinsey, say that executives around the world recognise the potential for using technology in health.[62] Over the past decade, many hospitals have invested heavily in e-health programs. Most have delivered only a modest return, as measured by higher care quality, greater efficiency or better patient outcomes. In some cases, e-health projects have been cancelled or entirely revamped as a result.[63]

Stefan Biesdorf and Florian Niedermann from McKinsey say that the digitisation of healthcare initially followed a similar pattern to other industries, but is now lagging behind, perhaps due to the many myths that prevail. They suggest that digitisation in healthcare ought to begin with the example offered by Google and Facebook. These organisations first offered a limited core service to a small market segment, and then built additional services and capacity as their users developed trust and gained confidence.[64]

The Real Issue

I'm suggesting the real challenge is the pushback from forcing busy clinicians, who have other things on their minds, to input constantly changing data into computers.[65] The way forward is to provide computers with sensors so that they can automatically capture data from the natural flow of work. The next chapter explores what hospitals are trying to do, and what they should focus on instead.

Summary

- Whilst digitisation provides a common language for different systems to talk and communicate with each other, this must be orchestrated using internet and transfer protocols – without forcing clinicians to enter data into computers.

- We are already using RFID in our daily lives – PayPass, electronic travel passes, and e-tags on freeways are examples. RFID has connected more than 15 billion things and these connections exceed all other networked devices combined. These hidden sensors can contribute to greater usefulness of our phones.

- Executives around the world are aware of the usefulness of digitisation. e-health initiatives would be more readily adopted if there was focus on providing computers with sensors to automatically capture RFID data in the natural flow of work. This will let clinicians focus on their patients without distraction.

- Hospitals need to use technology to simplify the routine and difficult 'jobs to be done'. Simplification in other industries has enabled the adoption of new business models, products and services. Communication has to be orchestrated using the internet and transfer protocols, though this has to be done without requiring clinicians to input constantly changing data into computers.

3

What Hospitals Are Doing

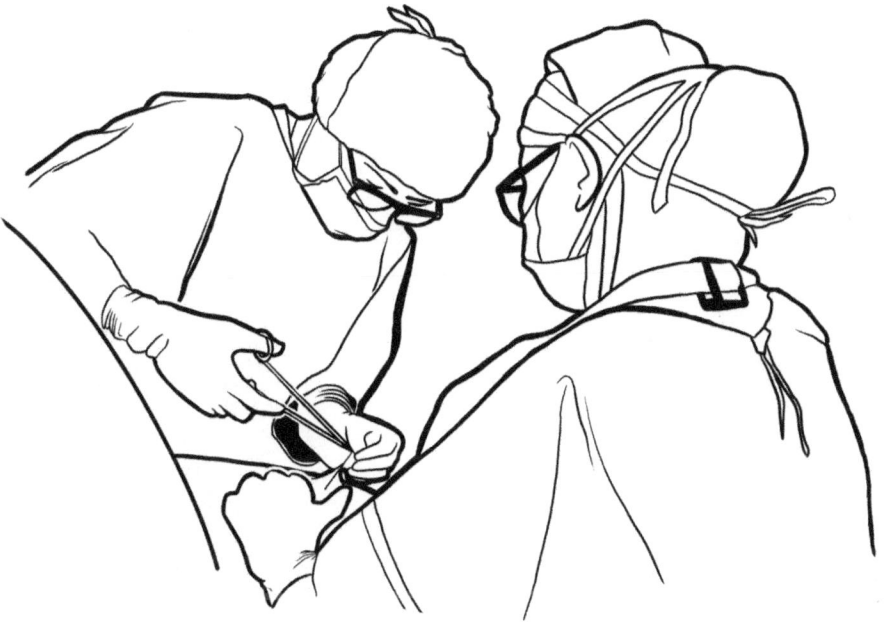

Hospital executives are acutely aware of the usefulness of digitisation and have embarked on digital journeys. However, they have had mixed results.[66] This may be because most healthcare providers believe they must offer a comprehensive platform as a prerequisite for offering value, when in fact all that is required is to start small and act fast.[67] This sentiment has been echoed by other healthcare specialists.[68] My own thinking, based on personal experience is that digital implementation often fails because clinicians are forced to update computers, a task that they do not see as part of their roles. I have suggested instead that we use context-aware computers with sensors to input data.

Clayton Christensen and his co-authors identified a pervasive pattern in every established industry transformed through disruption. The energies, talents, and resources of established organisations are focused on their most demanding applications, products, and services. This is because most profits are made from these products and services.

However, if the simpler problems are solved first, technological enablers are allowed to gain a foothold. They can then progressively displace old high-cost applications, products and services. For example, consider the experience with Uber. We hail our ride on a mobile device. We track our driver moving towards us and know how long we've got to wait for the pickup. We can estimate how long the ride to our destination will take and even know what it will cost. Then we exit our ride without having to touch our wallets.

I call the process living in a touch-to-know world.[69] In hospitals, such seamless use of technology has not yet been used for the many jobs that need to be 'done' repetitively and with difficulty. Hospitals remain focused on the large, complex tasks that require huge investments in learning new skills and changing the way that jobs are done. This distracts people from their primary tasks and raises resistance.[70]

This is not specific to the medical industry. Kevin Ashton believes that people in general focus digitisation on solving complex and intellectual problems when computers could also be used to tackle simpler problems, like finding lipstick on store shelves. This approach would have tremendous outcomes for fast-moving consumable goods. The huge potential for technology to change behaviour and outcomes is often missed.

The Potential of Technology to Change Behaviour and Outcomes

Steven Johnson beautifully encapsulates this idea with his article published in *The Guardian* entitled, 'Recognising the True Potential of Technology to Change Behaviour'.

He writes that technology could be successful in changing behaviours that decades of campaigns and legislation have failed to change. He suggests that with self-tracking devices being used by many of us and with the Internet of Things within easy reach, we ought to be more ambitious about creating opportunities to encourage, enable and empower sustainable behaviours. With self-tracking devices, information is harvested using sensors connected through the Internet of Things and returned to the end-user for an appropriate response.[71]

Erring on the Side of Caution

Besides investing in solving the most complex problems, healthcare is heavily invested in doing no harm. This focus, however, can be used to justify limitless expense and inefficiency, and to resist change. Hospitals want to be sure that new measures do no harm, and err on the side of caution by blocking any new innovation. Traditionally, healthcare leaders lobby for legislation and regulations to block any disruptive approach until its use can be certified 'good enough' to be used everywhere.[72] But while healthcare is seen to be cautious, adverse events kill many hundreds of thousands people each year.[73]

In 2016 there were potentially 27,000 avoidable deaths in Australia.[74] In mid-November 2016 Tim Kelsey, CEO of the Australian Digital Health Agency said that 'the number of people who die in Australia as a result of mis-prescribing inadvertently by clinicians is greater than the number of people who die from road traffic accidents.[75]

Clouded by Complexity

Clayton Christensen observes that hospitals are clouded by complexity. Many of the costs come from overhead activities rather than direct patient care, and hospitals are unable to appropriately allocate costs between the three separate functions they perform.

Firstly: hospitals function as 'solution shops' structured around the diagnosis and solving of unstructured problems. This is because most diseases share symptoms, and it is often difficult to identify the disease based solely on symptoms. Decision-making is done by experts who draw on their intuition and problem solving skills to diagnose causes. The popular TV programme *House* exemplifies such an approach. Atul Gawande, the well-known physician, author and TED speaker says, 'There is science in what we do, yes, but also habit, intuition, and sometimes plain old guessing. The gap between what we know and what we aim for persists. And this gap complicates everything we do'.[76]

Highly trained scientists and technicians amass information from imaging, pathology, monitoring equipment, and physical examination. Physicians intuitively develop a hypothesis of the causes and test their conjecture with the best treatment available until causes can be isolated and eliminated.

Secondly: hospitals are seen to function as value-adding processing businesses. In a value-added process, the perceived value of the process is much greater than the cost incurred. In hospitals, these can only be attributed to medical procedures that occur after a definitive diagnosis is made. These range from prescribing medicines, to nursing and even to surgery. The outcomes of such treatment can be fairly certain and definitive. It is here that Harvard Business Professor Steven Spear's 'Five Rules-in-Use' can be used in hospitals so that value-adding processes can be accurately costed.

- Rule 1 – Each step in a process must be completely specified so that the need for rework is eliminated. There's a clear go/no-go verification at the end of every process.

- Rule 2 – Never add value to a part that is defective. This means that you should never work on a part that is defective.

- Rule 3 – The sequence of steps that a part takes through the process must be completely specified as a series of one-to-one handoffs. The same worker always gives what he has done to the same worker to perform the next step. Any-worker to any-worker handoffs are not allowed.

- Rule 4 – Perform each step in your process the same way each and every time so as to test whether doing it this way will deliver the perfect result each time.

- Rule 5 – Never allow the cause of a problem to persist by working around it. We must change our methods whenever a faulty result occurs so that it cannot happen again.

I believe that in a hospital these rules are contentious. As Dave Gray, author of *The Connected Company*, says that services are contextual. They may require specialised knowledge or skills, but the value of a service lies in the interactions. It's not the end product that matters, as much as the experience.[77] It may be because of this and the current methods for costing that there is so much variation in the cost of surgery.[78] Steven J Stack, an emergency room physician, agrees that consistency, stability and predictability matters, but points out the job as imagined by administrators and the job as done in the ER are two different things.[79] He says that healthcare is often compared with the airline industry but there are striking differences:

- When was the last time we heard that only one pilot showed up for the flight and the airline allowed the airplane to take off?

- When was the last time we heard that the air crew didn't show up and the pilots said they would fly without the crew?

Yet in hospitals, in spite of staff shortages, equipment being down, drug shortages, lack of opioids, medazepam, paralytics, and normal saline among other things, the work has to go on. Sometimes when a physician needs to insert a chest tube in a hurry, he discovers someone in purchasing has decided to change the contract, so the clinician now has to learn how to use a new kit on the job. It's akin to asking airline pilots to fly a new passenger plane without any training.

Steven Stack clarifies that he sees the need for lean processes, but with taking out the non-value-add processes in hospitals, it is difficult because the way that the work is imagined is quite different from the way that the work is actually done.[80]

A link is provided here for you to see Steven Stack express his view at a conference:

https://www.youtube.com/watch?v=yQfZT2pdREM&t=271s

Finally: hospitals work as facilitated networks. These networks match service providers with consumers and vice versa. In hospitals, patients are matched with rehabilitation specialists, wellness educators, and even other patients who have gone through similar treatment and can learn from each other. Here, the focus is on wellness rather than illness. Many new-age businesses have grown to prominence by using facilitated networks. Many authors who have studied this phenomenon call this business model 'platform businesses'.[81]

Christensen believes that if these three processes can be separated, costing could be done accurately and each process would need to use different business models.[82]

This book contends that costing is difficult because the process for capturing costs is poorly designed. Hospitals need to use context-aware computers so that they can harvest data from the natural flow of work without distracting clinicians and nurses from their primary job – patient care – because healthcare is fundamentally a human endeavour.[83]

By using context-aware computers, some of the issues raised by Stack can be addressed through better communication engendered by the capabilities of touch-to-know technology.

What Hospitals Ought to Do

I have already suggested that all hospital items, information, media, and even events, ought to be represented digitally using UHF-RFID. This would enable information about items, events and their locations to be tracked and traced easily using any device with browsers connected to the internet.

With digitisation, an event may have passed, but the digital representation lives on. These digital representations could be used to fine-tune future events and improve business and safety processes.

What Is RFID?

There are several types and formats of RFID. In this book, I refer to passive radiofrequency identification. Radiofrequency identification (RFID) is the use of radio waves to read and capture information stored on an electronic tag that is attached to an object. A tag can be read from up to several feet away and does not need to be within direct line-of-sight of the reader to be tracked.

Quality of Data

Ian Robertson, a supply chain expert says, 'That there is nothing wrong with highlighting how RFID does not need line-of-sight to be tracked and traced. But, if this is the only difference that is highlighted then the many other benefits of the RFID/standards for RFID will remain undiscovered and probably unused.'[84]

Robertson goes on to say that the most important point about information at the operational level is that its quality is totally dependent upon the quality of the individual data it is made up from. An operation or hospital for that matter, which is managed on poor quality information is going to be poorly managed no matter how well the managers or workers perform their individual tasks. From my experience, this is what hospitals are labouring under.

Fred Kimball is making a similar observation when he asks, 'Is your inventory accuracy really as good as your auditor's report?'[85] He's calling out the difference between financial accuracy, which is about balancing the physical value of inventory with balance sheet reported values, as opposed to the actual accuracy of each line-item in inventory.

Item accuracy has implications for patient safety. Assume that two drugs are of similar value. If the shortage of one drug is compensated by the excess of the other, the financial value of the balance sheet doesn't change. In treatment, on the other hand, one drug cannot compensate for another. The outcome could be disasterous.

The Anatomy of an RFID System

It's hard to imagine that by attaching a small postage-sized RFID tag to items, hospitals can save millions and improve supply chain efficiencies by a minimum of 30%. There are other flow-on effects as well.

As mentioned earlier, an RFID system is comprised of four basic elements.

Tags	Antenna	Reader	Host Computer

Tags	Antenna	Reader	Host Computer
• Device made up of an electronic circuit and an integrated antenna • Portable memory • RF used to transfer data between the tag and the antenna • Read-only or read/write • Active or passive • Usually attached to specific items	• Receives and transmits the radio waves • Wireless data transfer	• Communicates with the tag via antenna • Interprets radio waves into digital information • Provides power supply to passive tags • Receives commands from application software	• Issues commands to reader and provides/receives data • Stores and evaluates obtained data • Links the transceiver to an application, e.g. ERP

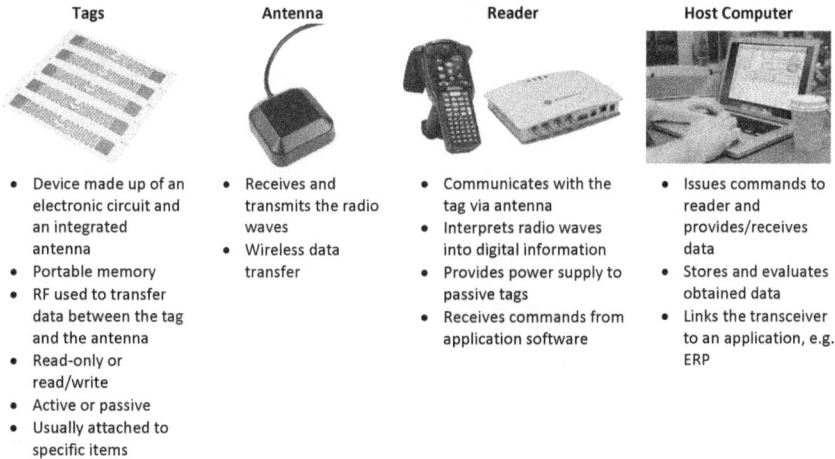

Four components of an RFID system

The tag is technically known as the transponder or receiver. This is a small chip, smaller than a grain of sand that can receive, store and return information when energised. The tag can read-only, write-only, or both read and write. This means that depending on the use, the tags can have relevant information written to the tag, read or even updated relating to events on its journey.

The antenna is an aerial attuned to receive and send electromagnetic waves.

Electromagnetic waves cover a wide spectrum of waves such as electric, radio, visible light, ultra-violet, X-rays, gamma rays, and cosmic rays. For the purpose of RFID, we are only interested in the radio-wave spectrum. In a tag, the antenna is attached to the tag's transponder, which is energised by radio waves. In hardware, it's attached to a reader to enable it to send and receive these radio waves.

The reader is an important hardware component since it communicates with the tag via the antenna, interprets the electronic waves converting them into digital information. This enables the reader to receive commands and communicate with the application software.

The computer sends and receives, or provides, data. It stores and evaluates the data received and links the RFID system to various other hospital systems.

In a retail setting, RFID tags may be attached to articles of clothing. When a sales assistant uses a handheld RFID reader to scan a shelf of jeans, they are able to differentiate between two pairs of jeans based upon the information stored on the RFID tag. Each pair will have its own serial number.

With one pass of the handheld RFID reader, the sales assistant can not only find a specific pair, but they can tell how many of each pair is on the shelf and which pairs need to be replenished, all without having to scan each individual item.

Kevin Ashton believed RFID was a prerequisite for the Internet of Things. He thought if all devices were tagged, computers could then manage, track, and inventory them.

Using UHF-RFID and the Internet of Things opens up many exciting possibilities for solving the jobs to be done in hospitals and could go a long way in addressing the problems faced with lack of time, space and margin.

Converting Hospital Losses into Gains

I want to focus on the centrality of the Internet of Things in assisting clinicians to focus on their patients and to provide them with 'error wisdom'[86] at their fingertips and reduce the impact of psychological and physical distance[87] that administrators experience when separated from the patient's side. This, in a sense, is what is so wonderful about the Internet of Things.

The Usefulness of the Internet of Things

Calum McClelland asks a series of simple and relevant questions that highlight the usefulness of the Internet of Things:[88]

1. 'How are you reading this post right now?'

- If it's hard copy, it likely started life as a digital representation on a computer that was later printed. If you're reading this on your desktop, your mobile phone, or even a tablet, then these devices are probably connected to the internet.

- He points out that this capability gives us all sorts of benefits that just weren't possible before. If you remember your mobile phone before it morphed into a smartphone, you would recall that you could only make and receive phone calls and, possibly, text messages. But now you can read any book, watch any movie, or listen to any song in the palm of your hand. And that's just to name a few of the incredible things your smartphone can do. The point is, connecting things to the internet yields many amazing benefits.

2. 'Why would we want to connect everything to the internet?'

- McClelland clarifies that when something is connected to the internet, it can do three things: it can collect and send information and it can receive information and act on it and it can also do both of these things. These three things have an exponential effect when they feed off each other.

- The awesome thing is it can do all these things without having super storage or supercomputing on your devices. All it requires is that your device is connected to the internet.

Collecting and Sending Information

Collecting and sending information is made easier using sensors to automate the data collecting process. These sensors come in a variety of shapes and sizes. They could be temperature sensors, motion sensors, moisture sensors, air quality sensors, or light sensors, just to name a few.[89] These sensors, along with a connection, allow us to automatically collect information from the environment which, in turn, allows us to make more intelligent decisions.

Just as our senses allow us to make sense of the world, sensors allow machines to make sense of the environment around them.[90]

Receiving and Acting on Information

We're all familiar with machines getting information and then following through with appropriate action. Our printers receive a document from our device and print it. Our car receives information from our electronic keys and releases the door lock. We use our credit cards to pay-and-go. In the background, our bank accounts are charged, the vendor's accounts are credited, the shop's inventory system is updated and possibly their computers reorder replenishments.

The real power of the internet arises when things can receive and send information and also act on predetermined instructions.

Doing Both

McClelland uses a farming example to demonstrate the usefulness of the Internet of Things. The sensors collect information about soil moisture to tell the farmer how much water the crops need. He points out that we don't actually need the farmer because the software can initiate action and the irrigation system can automatically turn on, based on how much moisture is in the soil.

This can be taken a step further. If the irrigation system receives information about the weather from its internet connection, it can also know based on the information received about the possibility of rain whether to water the crops or not.

All this siloed information from one farm, useful as it is, becomes even more useful when combined with information for all the other farms in the region. With the combined information from the region, algorithms can create incredible insights into how to make crops grow better. It's easy to see how such a capability could be useful in a hospital or group of hospitals in one geographic region.

The Electricity Metaphor

In his 2003 TED talk, Jeff Bezos compares the foray into the internet with the gold rush. There were telling similarities. With both, many people felt the compelling need to give up what they were doing to search instead for easy pickings. With both, there was a tremendous burn rate and great disappointment. With the gold rush, when the last nugget was taken, there was nothing left. It was over. With the internet, however, it was only the very beginning. If you really believed this, then there were still tremendous opportunities ahead. [91]

Electricity would perhaps be a better analogy. Both the internet and electricity require the transmission of power through thin parallel wires. They cover a broad range of industries and had a way of coordinating things in a fine granular manner. They allow for tremendous resilience. Electricity needs infrastructure for laying down the cables to bring light to homes. They weren't thinking of appliances when they wired the world. They weren't putting electricity into homes, they were putting lighting into the home. But once the light was introduced into homes, it also introduced the 'golden age of appliances'.

Like electricity, the internet required cables, but the infrastructure was already there. The internet sat above all the electrical infrastructure. Evan Andrews, author for the *Inside History* newsletter, says that the online world took on a more recognisable form in 1990 when computer scientist Tim Berners-Lee invented the World Wide Web. While it's often confused with the internet itself, the web is actually just the most common means of accessing data online in the form of websites and hyperlinks. The web helped popularise the internet among the public, and it served as a crucial step in developing the vast trove of information that most of us now access on a daily basis.[92]

Bezos ended his talk with a quote from the 1917 Sears' advertisement that said, 'Use your electricity for more than light…' Bezos thought that opportunities for using the internet was like when electricity was first introduced into the home at the very early stages of innovation and development.

Today, the internet, along with the innovative use of sensors built on the electricity infrastructure, gives us the ability to manage business dynamics as never before. Google, Apple, Facebook, Amazon and a host of other companies have learnt to digitise their marketplaces with a new business model – platforms.

Platforms

A platform is a marketplace that uncouples the traditional cost and profit structures by not owning the means of production. A platform treats everyone – those that consume the product and those that produce the products – as customers.

After incurring the initial cost of creating a platform, the cost to serve additional customers falls close to zero. Platforms earn income by capturing a portion of the value they create from encouraging consistent, efficient and ongoing transactions.

Hospitals have all the necessary ingredients in place to be combined into a unified platform. When they stand alone, like the example that Calum McClelland drew of the individual farm, it could be valuable, but if this information was pooled across all hospitals in a common geographic location it would have momentous value. It would reduce hospital costs, improve margins and improve patient safety across the whole industry.

That's why Jonathan Bush, co-founder and former chief executive officer of Athenahealth, says that Google, Microsoft, Facebook, and loads of smaller companies keep prowling in the vicinity, looking for their niche. These companies, he adds, have chosen a rough road. In their attempts to take control of the business opportunities offered by healthcare, they've been battered and bruised.[93]

Gaining a Foothold in Healthcare

I believe that for businesses outside health to make in-roads into healthcare is difficult because of the many workarounds that abound in hospitals. These are the hidden hazards in making a margin. The numbers that they see are only a partial and incorrect view of what happens at the working interface.[94] This is what Ian Robertson refers to when he enunciates his thoughts about the accuracy of information.[95]

It will only be possible to run a profitable hospital if we digitise all materials, information and events to help provide accurate data. With RFID, the information can be automatically harvested from the natural flow of work and pushed to the internet for sharing. Only then will the psychological and physical distance between administrators, clinicians, and patients in a hospital be removed to provide information that can be responded to appropriately.

Response to Physicians

Jonathan Bush points out that in the healthcare economy, doctors have more power than hospitals.[96] In a market focused on establishing long-term relationships with patients, doctors hold the cards. And, as Fred Lee points out that with private care, hospitals don't have patients, physicians do.[97] The hospital cares for physicians' patients. Hence, it's the doctor who is the customer. However, this is not contrary to the view that the patient must be the centre of focus.

Martin Bowles, previously Secretary for the Department of Health, says when we speak of healthcare we usually mean hospitals.[98] This is because whilst more than 90% of healthcare occurs outside the hospital, hospitals account for the major expenditure in the health budget. The out-of-hospital costs that Bowles referred to are probably the costs incurred for the treatment of chronic disease. These are payments for the care of those with behaviour-dependent diseases that have deferred consequences. The issue here is to facilitate behaviour change.[99] Perhaps medication prompters and fitness apps can assist in this.

Electronic Medical Records

The push by governments to further the cause of e-health records doesn't always happen. Each year in Australian hospitals 546,544 patients leave worse off than when they were admitted.[100] This is not because of their illness, this is because clinicians and nurses make preventable errors in the course of treatment.

For hospitals to improve patient safety, they must provide clinicians and nurses with contextual prompts to help them locate the items they need and help them to complete tasks. James Reason calls this providing clinicians with 'error wisdom' at the sharp end.[101]

Providing Timely Prompts

Let's look at an app that's already on the market that helps patients to take their prescription medications. Studies have shown that only 50 percent of patients take their medication regularly as prescribed by their physicians.[102]

MyTherapy is a medication prompter that reminds the user when it's time to take their medication and sends the user and their caregiver reminders if the medication has not been taken. Reports suggest the app has increased compliance of taking medication by 45 percent.

The app requires the patient to manually input information into the system to work. The information required includes medication name, dosage, time/schedule, duration and other relevant details pertaining to the medication.

In hospitals, an app like MyTherapy in its current format would require clinicians manually input information into the computer system and would be seen as yet another task to be performed.

However, the medication could be represented digitally by using UHF-RFID to identify the medication. Then data input could be automated and the medication tracked and traced by sensors. The app could then prompt clinicians if the medication was not taken and could also ensure that there are no other iatrogenic implications.[103]

Financial Consideration

Hospitals are in financial trouble due to the way that executives, nurses and clinicians respond to the perceived lack of time, space and materials[104]. Most workers in hospitals see these as limitations. If hospitals want to overcome these limitations, as I have suggested before, they can install touch-to-know capability in their environment. To do this they must first digitise the hospital supply chain.

Supply Chain Disruption

Supply chain disruption is the term that Christensen and his co-authors use to depict the way that major pharmaceutical and medical device companies are losing market share to smaller business by outsourcing their supply chains.[105] Many large pharmaceutical and medical device companies that have long dominated the business arena have begun to get out of their least profitable activities and concentrate on increasing their profitability by investing in their most profitable products. The warehousing and distribution of goods is one such activity.

When dominant pharmaceutical businesses outsource their warehousing and distribution to third party warehousing and transportation companies, they inadvertently weaken their hold on the market. The third party warehousing and distribution businesses gradually take on more and more of the value-adding activities that the leaders outsource until they can eventually dominate large segments of the markets themselves. This leads to a level playing field over time.

Airbnb and Uber have shown us that access to other peoples' assets (with permission) is more important than owning the assets themselves. Their business model helps people utilise their time, space and materials more appropriately[106]. Hospitals could quite easily do the same with a small investment in technology or by partnering with a third party logistics provider by digitising product information on the items themselves. If hospitals did this, then with the use of appropriate apps they could 'hail' the items they needed from the nearest locations.

Why should hospitals curate the use of high-cost medical devices and pharmaceutical drugs when physicians bring patients to hospitals? Why not instead earn brokerage from matching product with physicians?

In many network business models, the dependency among users[107] is the main product delivered[108]. This could be similar to Amazon's marketplace infrastructure. It's even likely, if this 'job to be done' is solved, Google, Microsoft, Facebook, and loads of smaller companies may as yet be able to find footholds in healthcare.

Summary

- Hospital executives have embarked on ambitious digital journeys but have had mixed results to date. This may be because they don't start small and move quickly enough, believing instead that they must offer a platform of services that are comprehensive from the beginning.

- When hospitals focus on the complex time-consuming challenges, it causes unnecessary distraction and pushback from users. Yet, technology has the ability to change behaviour where campaigns and legislation have failed, if jobs to be done are simplified and made more convenient.

- Hospital decision-making is restrained because the process of gathering data is too manual. Data gathering is done by people focused on other tasks and produces inaccurate or missing information. RFID, supported by access to the internet, makes it possible to obtain accurate and dependable data and overcomes the limitations that hospitals face.

- RFID supported by the internet also makes it possible to track and trace all materials used and prevents the many workarounds that contribute to added costs and waste and promotes patient safety. The ability to track and trace materials make it possible to promote the use of touch-to-know apps.

- RFID and IoT make it possible for hospitals to use supply chain disruption and adopt a platform business model. This aligns physicians and hospital interest for the benefit of patients.

4

Automating ERP Data Entry

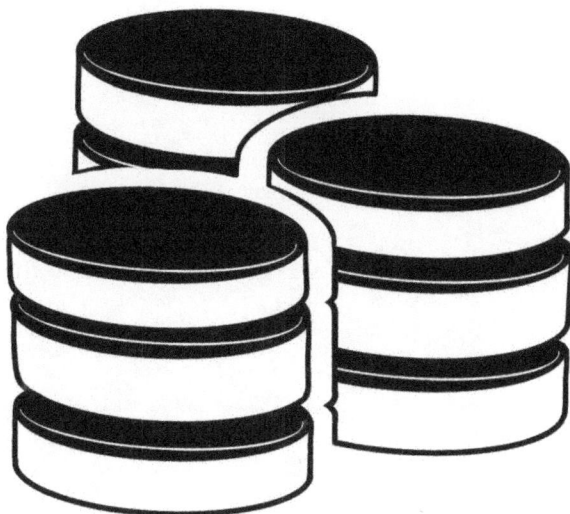

ERP Systems

In 1999 I was invited to join a small select team to implement J D Edwards an ERP System at Cabrini Health. J D Edwards is a relational database. I soon realised that with relational databases, instead of the end user's needs driving the requirements for the database, it was the other way around. The database dictated how end-users had to work. A constant question from the nurses and clinicians was, 'Why do we have to work for JDE? Why can't JDE work for us?'

Since 1999 the situation has worsened. Dave McComb who writes about semantics in computing systems and data-centricity says that we've reached a turning point in the way we manage entreprise information. The amount of data available is doubling each year, but [for most of us] our ability to use it effectively decreases.[109] His sentiments are echoed by Arkady Maydanchik who wrote about data quality as early as 2007.[110]

Maydanchik says that although information systems get better, data quality deteriorates. He writes that high quality data combined with effective technology is a great asset, but poor quality data combined with effective technology is a great liability.[111]

Data quality does not improve by itself or as a result of general IT advancement. Maydanchick's diagram following shows how internal and external sources can affect data quality negatively unless the process is sufficiently resourced.

In hospitals the logic for getting physicians and clinicians to manually input data into computers is questionable. Their primary focus is elsewhere.

In my experience, asking people focussed on other things is designed to seed incorrect information into the system. This insight has been validated by experts on human error.[112]

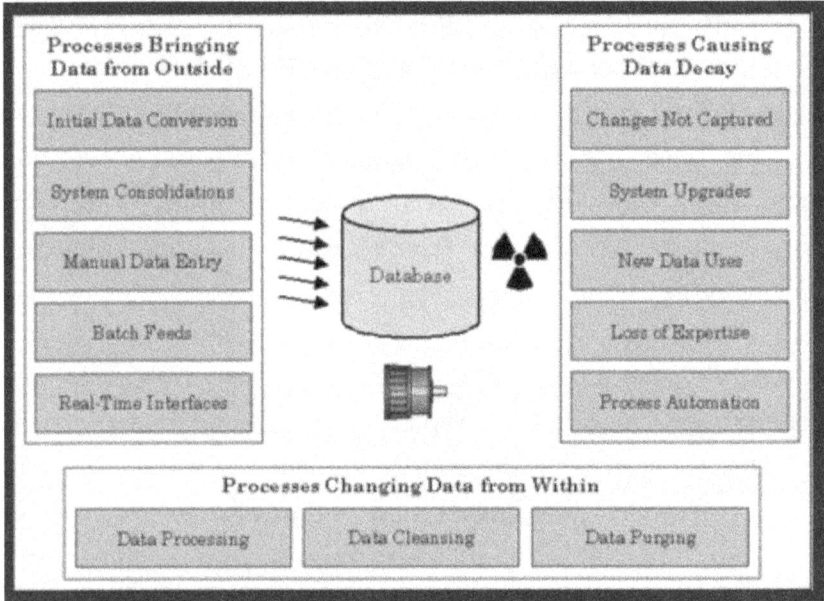

Processes Bringing Data from Outside	Processes Causing Data Decay
Initial Data Conversion	Changes Not Captured
System Consolidations	System Upgrades
Manual Data Entry	New Data Uses
Batch Feeds	Loss of Expertise
Real-Time Interfaces	Process Automation

Database

Processes Changing Data from Within		
Data Processing	Data Cleansing	Data Purging

Self-sufficient Computers

The irony is that this situation need not persist. In the previous chapter, I pointed out that Kevin Ashton has already solved the problem of inputting data into computers without human intervention.[113]

Ashton's insight was that people saw computers as brains without sensors. The expectation was that humans, busy doing other things, had to provide the input. He solved this problem by providing computers with sensors so that they could sense the environment around them for themselves without the need for human input.

In today's world, this has become even easier. As I have pointed out before, our smart phones are context-aware devices that could be used as input devices for computers in special circumstances.

A Mindset Problem

Dave McComb says that executives suffer from a mindset problem.[114] He blames the current woes on a firmly entrenched mindset. As a technology consultant, he believes that executives are addicted to their points of view. The more they struggle with their systems the more they invest and the more stuck they become.

They believe that software is expensive and difficult to implement because that's the way it's always been. This would not be the case if, like in the automotive industry, software adopted lean manufacturing principles to dramatically improve productivity and quality. He acknowledges that a few 21st century companies are successfully adopting such an approach.[115]

Werner Vogels, VP & CTO of Amazon cites examples from Amazon, Airbnb and other new age companies that successfully do this. He says that in the past the only database choice for many entreprises was a relational database and no matter the shape or function of the data in the application, the data was modelled as relational.[116]

With relational databases, instead of the use-case driving the requirements for the database, it was the other way around. The database was driving the data model for the applicaion use case.

Vogels' point is that not all application data models or use cases match the relational model but this needen't be a limitation. Relational databases still provide utility are scalable and can provide high performance. It is when entreprise tries to use relational databases beyond their intended purpose that we have efficiency issues. He believes that developers ought to build databases that match the end-users needs, are well architected and can scale effectively.

With the customer in mind, Amazon has been able to build multiple databases and data models within the same application.

Vogle says that seldom can one database fit the needs of multiple distinct use cases. The days of the one-size-fits-all monolithic database are behind us, and developers are now building highly distributed applications using a multitude of purpose-built databases.

Developers are doing what they do best: breaking complex applications into smaller pieces and then picking the best tool to solve each problem. The best tool for a job usually differs by use case.

Amazon has, as have other software companies, been able to build and use several types of databases in specific applications for their customers. These applications include databases that are:

- Relational
- Key-value
- Document
- Graph
- In-memory, and
- Search

The Way Out of the Quagmire

McComb calls the current entreprise bind a quagmire.[117] McComb's approach is to build a data-centric entreprise where all application functionality is based on a single, simple, extensible data model.[118] He suggests that the problem is not a technological one. He suggests that it's to see the landscape and the problem differently and then having the courage and discppline to change course. McComb sees a parallel between the industrial revolution when electricity eventually displaced steam.

It was not technology that slowed the transition, it was resistance from a tight-knit network of experts who reinforced the status quo. The situation is the same today when managers in charge of many direct reports, and very large budgets are not motivated to reduce the size and importance of their empires.

Building a data-centric architecture has all the same properties as a building has shells. [119] The foundation of a data-centric architecture is based on enduring business themes. These are the core concepts that remain constant over decades or longer. The things that are layered on this foundation can change more rapidly without disturbing the core.

The inclusion of all data types

Dave McComb says that the data-centric approach provides an answer to one of the most vexing problems in the entreprise information system space:[120] the integration of structured and unstructured data.

Werner Vogles says that the world is changing and the categories of nonrelational databases continue to grow. Developers are building highly distributed and decopupled applications to serve these needs.[121]

A data model with several databases

Having a single data model does not imply having a single database. In most installations, there will be many databases that conform to the core model. The architecture to support the data-centric model will ensure that the different databases can be queried to obtain acombined result. The single-core model provides the ability to execute queries.

McComb calls these federated queries. A federated query is one where it is distributed to multiple databases, each of which solves a portion of the problem, and then the results are combined.

The key takeaway is that these federated queries can include databases that were loaded directly into the data-centric model, as well as existing legacy databases that have been mapped to the data-centric model. This approach allows organisations to build their own enterprise app store.

The Entreprise App Store

Suggesting a touch-to-know environment is premised on answering the question that is uppermost in our minds. 'If we can have app functionality and convenience in our personal lives, why can't we have the same functionality in our working environment?'

The short answer is that apps in our personal lives have very low data integration demands. Whatever little integration required is done by the end user themselves. For instance, the user might load all their contacts into an app. This is really personal ad hoc integration.

Such apps cannot manage inventory, process orders, settle invoices and perform many other complex functions that an enterprise routinely performs.

However, if the entreprise apps are built from an entreprise's shared data model, everything the app requires will come from the entreprise's data model and the results of the actions taken on the app will be returned to the shared model.

Using this approach, entreprises can have apps on mobile devices that manage inventory, process orders, settle invoices and perform many other complex functions that are required routinenly in organisations. The additional benefit as apps are best suited to single function tasks is that data cleansing becomes easier.

By default, it becomes a continuous improvement project in itself and encourages every user to correct misinformation as they use these entreprise apps.

The economics

The apps that we use in our personal lives are purchased for less than $1 in most instances. The low price is justified because of the number of downloads for personal apps. This will not be the case for bespoke apps used by organisations. The low volume of specialised users would demand a higher cost. But when seen in the context of savings, such apps would generate the return on investment that would justify the higher costs.

Taylor Pearson, a well-known author, has written a wonderful post on why organisations and states don't avail of valuable opportunities. It is based on the concept of legibility. He builds his insight on the seminal work of James Scott the author of 'Seeing Like a State'.[122] Pearson's summary is that "we assume that only what we can measure is real and everything that is real can be measured."

Pearson's point is that what cannot be measured – the illegible margin can be immense. The smartphone boom has proved this. But this is not limited to smartphones. The discovery of margin in other areas also has a lot of profit potential. I believe this is particularly pertinent to hospitals.

Building the Database

Stan Geiger says that databases do not build themselves. However, data modelling can help design and build efficient, highly performing, and relevant databases.[123]

Creating a touch-to-know environment involves building peripheral databases to automate data input into hospital ERP systems. It uses Mandanchick's concept that foreign keys[key-values] are the glue that holds the database together. Without foreign keys, the data is like leaves covering the ground in the fall – you know that each leaf fell from one of the trees, but it is impossible to say from which one.

In hospitals complex tasks can be broken into smaller tasks that will allow apps to automatically consume and update data. This approach can be used for:

- Mobile first materials management – automates receiving, storage, distribution and reordering of materials seamlessly.

- Procedure costing that is currently a tedious and error prone process.

- Preferece card management – automatic synchronisation of procedure cards, preference cards, guided picking and returns of unused items to the store.

- Prosthetic item management – automates rebate code updates and claims management for items consumed.

- Consignment stock management – automates consignment counts in real time.

- Data cleansing – provides federated queries across several databases and updates information automatically.

Summary

In this chapter, I suggest that we follow Kevin Ashton's lead and provide ERP systems with sensors to gather information from the context in which they are being used instead of having nurses and clinicians input data into computers.

I have suggested that this can be done by breaking complex tasks into simpler components and use entreprise apps to gather and disseminate the neccessar information. Touch to Know has developed such apps to assist with internal hospital supply functions.

In the next chapter, I explain how this has implications for good clinical practise.

5

Using Technology to Simplify Patient Safety

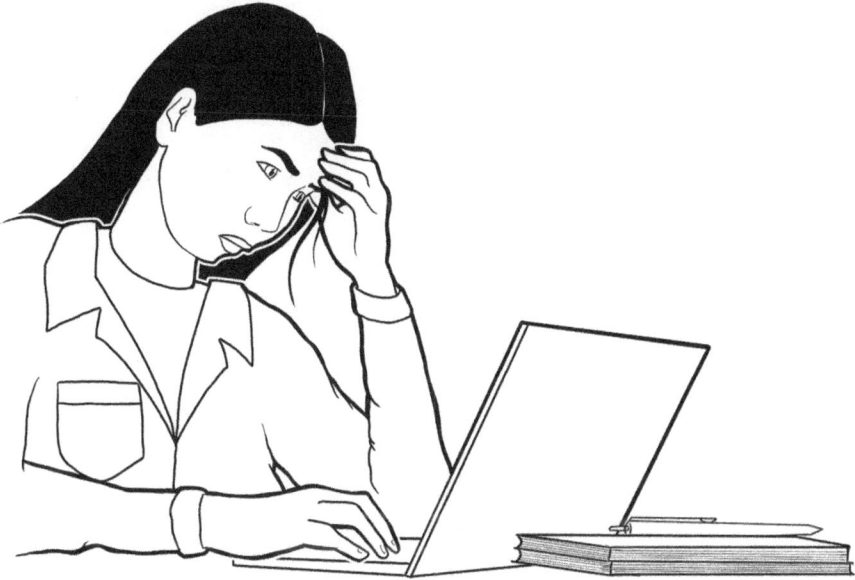

I began this book by lamenting that touch-to-know capability had not reached hospitals. I thought that such human–computer interaction could help in preventing adverse events in hospitals and also improve hospital margins. I observed that hospitals were not averse to using technology; however, they were keen on tackling the bigger and more complex problems of treatment rather than focusing on simplifying mundane everyday tasks[124] that got in the way of operational efficiency. These tasks were too small to gain the attention of management, though they still accounted for a fifth of a nurse's working day.[125]

I expressed that hospital executives had not realised that by simplifying tasks, technology had more potential to change thinking and behaviours than years of campaigning and legislation.[126] Smartphones have become an integral part of our lives. With apps on our smartphones, we perform previously tedious jobs, easily and conveniently. Without apps, these tedious jobs may not have been performed at all.

In Chapter 3, I highlighted that the emotional aspects of jobs in hospitals elicited defensive behaviour that derailed many hospital processes. I explained that UHF-RFID was the missing link in the suite of technologies that hospitals needed in order to use apps to make jobs more convenient and seamless to perform. With these apps, we could easily manage the thousands of moveable assets and medical consumables that distracted clinicians from focusing fully on patient care.

Technology for Patient Safety

B J Fogg was one of the first scientists to realise that computers could be used as persuasive tools.[127] In 1997, during his final year as a doctoral student, Fogg spoke at a conference in Atlanta on how computers might be used to influence the behaviours of their users. He noted that interactive technologies were no longer just tools for work – they had become part of our everyday lives. We used them to manage finances, study and even to stay healthy.

Yet, computer scientists were still focusing on the machines they were making rather than on the people that were using them.

Fogg presented the results of a simple experiment that he had run at Stanford, which showed that people spent longer on tasks if they were working on a computer they felt had previously been helpful to them. In other words, their interaction with computers followed the same rules of reciprocity that psychologists identified in social life. The significance of this finding was that computer applications could be designed to use the rules of psychology in order to get people to do things they might not otherwise do.

Fogg founded the Behaviour Design Lab at Stanford University to help innovators assist people to use computers more effectively using his models and methods of behaviour design.[128] Behaviour design is now embedded into the invisible operating system of our everyday lives. The emails that induce us to buy right away, the apps and games that rivet our attention, the online forms that nudge us towards one decision over another are all designed to influence our behaviour[129]. One of the cornerstones of Fogg's thinking is his behaviour model.

For somebody to do something, three things must happen at once. The person must want to do it, they must be able to do it, and they must be prompted to do it. In other words, there must be a timely call to action. This can be translated to motivation, ability, and a context sensitive prompt. If any of these three things are missing, then the behaviour is likely to fail.

The model is being explained in the context of nursing and patient safety. The model is a conceptual representation, so the two axes have no measurements. Using the model, we can immediately see that when motivation is high we can ask people to perform harder tasks, but when motivation is low, we can only get them to perform easier tasks.

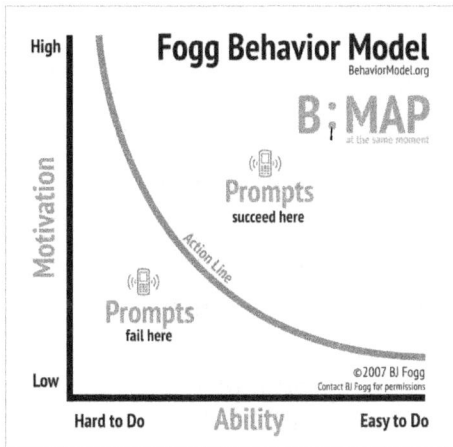

The Fogg Behaviour Model

The Action Line

The action line, or the slippery slope of success as Fogg has sometimes called it, does not touch either axis on the behaviour model above. This is because if the task is hard, people can get frustrated. Or if the task is easy to do, and they're not motivated to do it, they can get annoyed if constantly asked to perform such tasks.

Fogg suggests that frustrations are more fixable than an annoyance. When we want people to do something, our first instinct is to try to increase their motivation. Sometimes this may work; however, increasing motivation is a difficult undertaking because different people are motivated by different things. Fogg says, 'You can't get people to do something they don't want to do.' The better route to take is to make the task easier to do and then it is more likely they will take action.

Prompts

When motivation is sufficiently high, or the task is easy to do, people become responsive to prompts, such as the vibration of a phone. The key is to design the prompt to occur in a context-sensitive manner just when people are most eager to take action.

Seen in this light, the focus must be on simplifying tasks and then ensuring that there is a context-sensitive call for action. This route will ensure easier success. If the prompt occurs when we are attending to something that we cannot stop, such as when a nurse is resuscitating a patient, the prompt will fail.

On the other hand, if the prompt is missing completely, a nurse may not perform a task at all. For example, nurses are often asked to return telephone calls. These requests are usually made when they are in the midst of performing a complex and time-consuming job, a job that may take 30 to 35 minutes to complete. The calls may never be returned because of the lack of contextual prompts when the job is completed.

Contextual Prompts

Contextual prompts are useful if we can find users at the moment when they're most able to take action. If they're prompted to do something they don't like, they probably won't do it. But if they're prompted to do something they want to do, they'd probably comply and love it. The emotional satisfaction is likely to make people feel successful and reinforces the need to continue such activity and possibly to 'show and tell' others about it too.

Show and Tell

Fogg built his theories on behaviour design and influence before he realised how social platforms and network effects could amplify the impact of the 'show and tell' effect.[130] In his keynote address at the Persuasive Technology Conference in 2008, he shared his thoughts about 'mass interpersonal persuasion'. He realised that social media apps could reach deep into our motivations to share information with friends and peers. Their responses prompted each person to share the information with their networks, and with such sharing the impact could quickly become huge.[131] Sharing introduces a degree of variability. We don't know in advance what will be shared and with what frequency.

The Principle of Variable Rewards

One of Fogg's alumni, Nir Eyal, wrote a hugely popular book aimed at teaching tech entrepreneurs how to build apps that could successfully engage their target audiences. Eyal's approach focuses on the variability of the reward and the anticipation of satisfaction that keeps people coming back for more to become psychologically hooked into touching and scrolling on their phones constantly.

How Is This Relevant to Hospitals?

Hospitals have several challenges. In this book previously, I have identified ten, but have focused on two here:

- Patient safety
- The need for hospitals to contain costs

Both challenges arise because of human behaviour and both can be solved by using the same technology infrastructure.

Patient Safety

Whilst the vast majority of errors are inconsequential and go unnoticed, in certain circumstances, they combine to produce an adverse incident. These errors do not necessarily equate to incompetence, but we have a duty of care to change the conditions under which people work to make errors less likely and more easily recoverable.[132]

One of the biggest causes of error is the nature of the tasks and the procedures that require people to behave in unnatural ways, such as manually recording the many items used in surgery while trying to pay attention to the patient on the table.[133] See also Steven Stack's comments on multi-tasking in Chapter 2.[134] Providing contextual-prompts after interruptions can assist to reduce errors.

Containing Costs

Measurement is important. But looking at results tells us little about the causes of these results, especially if the numbers gathered are based on a poorly designed process.[135] I refer here to my experience of using a 'check-out' process for items consumed in the operating suite and anecdotal reporting about the mistakes made using barcode scanning.

Hospitals must use context-aware computers to gather data from the natural flow of work without distracting users from their primary tasks. This can be done by attaching UHF-RFID tags to all materials used in hospitals. The costing details can be automatically produced when packaging is discarded into smart bins.

Context-Aware Computers

As Kevin Ashton discovered in 1997, the ability for computers to detect unstocked shelves of lipstick was a symptom of one of the world's biggest problems: computers were brains without senses.[136] Computers processed data that people entered. And if the inputs were incorrect, the management information provided was likewise inaccurate.

If hospitals used context-aware computers with UHF-RFID tags for materials, then clinicians could receive context-aware prompts from apps that had access to this data, and hospital executives could also get accurate procedure costs to make better decisions.

Network effects provided by such a system open up other social dimensions to influence the hospital community. This requires, what has now come to be known as social-platforms. Hospitals could use and build on their own internal social-platform.

Summary

- B J Fogg was one of the first computer scientists to realise that computers could be used to persuade and influence people to lead better lives. He realised that computer scientists were focused on their machines, making them better, instead of being focused on the people that used their tools.

- A central tenet of Fogg's work is that three things must coincide at the same moment. People must want to do something, they must have the ability to take action, and there must be a prompt to call them to take action. If any of these three things are missing the behaviour does not take place. Fogg suggests that the key to designing a prompt is for it to occur just when people are most eager to take action.

- One of the drivers of behaviour is people feeling successful when they take action and wanting to share their successes with others. Networked systems our social connection can spread the word of our successes. The significance of this for hospitals is: (1) Technology can provide contextual prompts for patient safety; (2) technology provides accurate cost and inventory information for better decision-making; and (3) with the ability to use mass interpersonal influence, hospitals can build their own internal social-platform for information sharing.

6

Context-Aware Apps

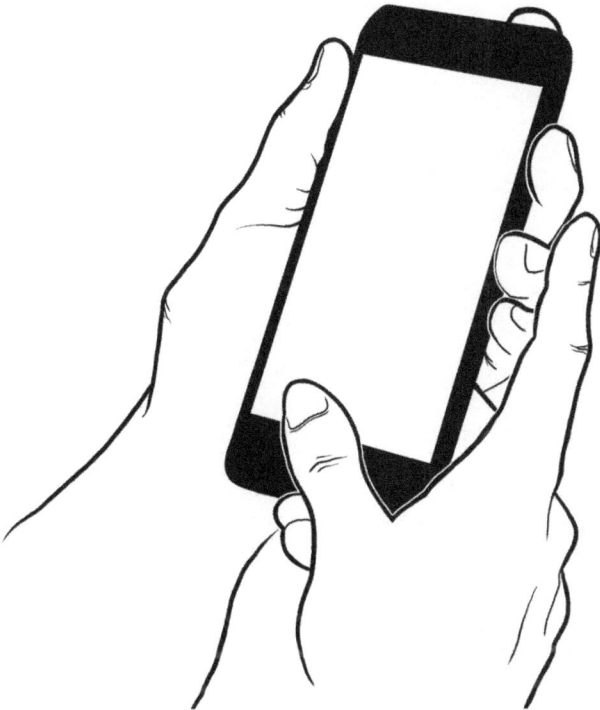

In Chapter 5, I expressed that B J Fogg was one of the first scientists to realise that computers could be used to positively influence the behaviour of people.137 Most computer scientists focused on the functioning of their machines rather than on the people that used their machines. Fogg realised that for successful behaviour to occur, people need to be motivated, have the ability to perform the behaviour and need to be prompted.138 All three elements need to be present at the same moment for a behaviour to occur. Most often for motivated people, behaviours do not occur because a prompt is missing at the time that the behaviour is required. In this chapter, we focus on the provision of 'context-aware' prompts. These are prompts that we receive from smartphones and other smart devices whilst performing tasks without altering the users normal schedule.

Generally, context-awareness is the ability of smartphones and other mobile devices to sense their physical surroundings and adapt to the environment. For instance, our smartphones react to the ambient light and adjust the screen brightness for optimal readability. As soon as the user touches the phone, the phone is activated and configures a setting to ensure the best possible user experience given the environment.

Context-aware apps have been around since the 1990s. They have taken off because of the widespread use of smartphones embedded with location service receivers (GPS). These are one of many sensors now bundled with smartphones[139]. Manisha Priyadarshini[140] from Fossbytes, an Indian technology media company, has identified sixteen different sensors used in smartphones. The use of these sensors opens up a whole new set of services that mobile phone app developers can now offer that do not need people to enter information, because the information is detected and input by the sensors themselves.

Find-My-Phone

Recently I had the opportunity to use an app that I hadn't tried before. My phone has a protective magnetic case so that it can be attached to the dashboard when I'm driving. One Sunday morning, distracted by buckling grandchildren into their seats before leaving home, I left the phone on the roof of the car. Later in the day, try as I might, I couldn't find my phone. As a last resort, I used the Find-My-Phone app on my computer. My phone was pinpointed on a GPS map, six kilometres away in Mornington. I hadn't even been to Mornington that day!

When I drove there, I discovered that I'd arrived at the Mornington Police Station. Somebody had found the phone, which had fallen on the road, and taken the trouble to leave it at the police station for collection. Although the screen was shattered, the phone was still working.

To find my phone, all I had to do was to fire up the app. The app had all my personal data, and the sensors on the phone provided the information required to locate it on a GPS map.

Proof of Delivery

Gonçalo Veiga cites an example of a context-aware app that his organisation had been asked to develop for a delivery company. The app was developed for PDA use. When the driver of a delivery truck parks at a client organisation to make a delivery, immediately the driver touches the PDA, the app instantly refreshes the screen with the package information for that location.

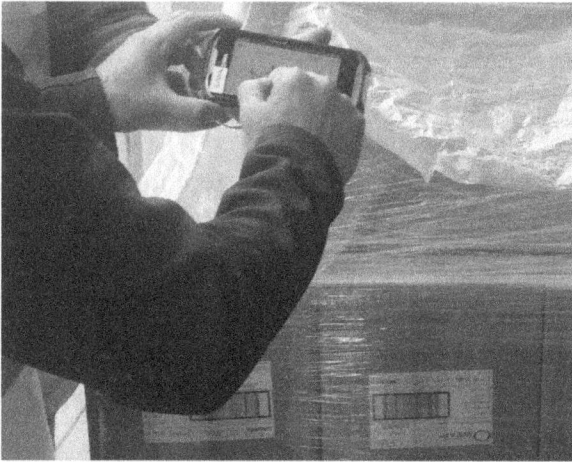
PDA being refreshed for item & location

As the driver approaches the back of the truck, the device communicates with the back door of the truck. The door unlocks, a green light indicates where the package is stored in the truck. When the package is dropped off on the client's loading dock, a delivery note is printed for attachment to the parcel. The delivery note is time-stamped to indicate the time of delivery. The driver gets back into his truck and drives off for his next drop-off.

Internally, in hospitals, no such apps are being used. Thousands of parcels are delivered to clinicians daily, yet the process is manual, onerous and error-prone. Anita Tucker, a researcher in hospital efficiencies, found that nurses spend a fifth of their working day looking for stock or supplies, an activity that takes them away from their patients.[141]

Context-Aware Apps for Hospitals

Context-awareness can dramatically improve workflows in hospitals by preventing clinical errors and by pre-empting patient falls. A major reason for human error is the poor design of work, and hospital distractions[142]. Each year in Australian hospitals, as many as 546,544 patients leave hospital worse off than when they were admitted[143]. In the financial year 2015–16, approximately 34,000 falls occurred in Australian hospitals and approximately 37% of these falls resulting in patient death.[144]

Unlike mobile apps that use machine-generated information, most processes in hospitals, still require clinicians to input constantly changing data into computers. This adds to the burden of work to be performed. If hospitals used context-aware devices bundled with sensors, these devices could sense, adapt, understand, and input machine generated data for clinicians.

For instance, if nurses have to administer medication to patients, they have to record this information on their charts by writing or scanning barcodes. However, by using context-aware sensors, most changing information could be machine generated and this would eliminate the need for manual record keeping.

For example, when I'd lost my phone and then retrieved it, I was able to retrace my phone's journey on a driving app on the phone. I found that the phone had been picked up on a cobbled bridge 600 metres away from my home then was driven to the Mornington Police Station, 12 minutes away. It remained at the police station for 3 hours before I picked it up. It had been rung three times but was left unanswered at the police station. All this information had been gathered by the phone seamlessly using sensors. I hadn't input any of the data into the device myself.

The Capability to Sense

Smartphones, with the many sensors bundled in them, have the ability to receive inputs from the environment or the device itself.[145] They can receive these inputs either explicitly or implicitly. The phone continues to process information as it is used, and apps on the phone are activated when particular environmental conditions are met. When activated, the phone prompts the user by alarms, pings, or vibrations, drawing attention to the environmental context.

The Capability to Adapt

The context-awareness arises because sensors detect changes and the ability to adapt arises from the use of algorithms to discern what the changes in time, location, speed, proximity or any other explicitly declared values mean in a given context. However, to be useful in hospitals, phones in the hands of clinicians must be able to receive inputs from sensors on the phone or in the hospital environment.

For instance, GPS does not always work well indoors. For location services to work indoors, phones must be able to receive input from sensors in the internal hospital environment.

Context-Awareness in Hospitals

The missing link in hospitals is the lack of sensors and limited use of RFID for the thousands of materials, moveable assets, and patient and staff name tags. Using sensors in these items enables communication with clinicians' smartphones or clinical specific devices. Merely by touching the screens on their phones or the devices, clinicians could more adequately manage things and communicate with people around them.

By receiving prompts on touchscreens, information becomes physical.[146] The table below shows how sensors in smartphones and materials can provide information to assist clinicians to avoid error and keep patients safe:[147]

Sensors	Prompts for action
Accelerometers and gyroscopes detect movement, vibration and orientation. This gives the device the ability to tell how fast it is moving and the direction of travel. They can also identify the orientation of the device, facing upwards, downwards, horizontal or vertical and rotation.	When people are admitted to hospitals and aged-care facilities, they are screened for the propensity to fall. With the ability to detect small changes in position from devices worn by these people, algorithms could predict their intention to get up and move. Receiving prompts on the phone enables clinicians to prevent falls by providing assistance.
Magnetometers and proximity sensors provide magnetic orientation and nearness to objects.	Since GPS does not work indoors and if beacons or other indoor sensing hardware are not installed, algorithms using input from magnetometers and proximity sensors on smartphones can be used to create indoor maps using blue dot technology to help locate places, objects and people. In such instances, clinicians can use search functions to locate the objects or people they need.

Sensors	Prompts for action
Ambient light sensors enable the phone to adjust the screen brightness dependant on the brightness of the environment.	While hospitals and medical clinics already use ambient light sensors in pulse-oximeters and glucometers for blood testing, these are not communicated to smartphones. If the readings rise above or below acceptable parameters, prompts could be sent to clinicians' smartphones for action.
Capacitive sensors in screens allows them to act as an input device.	Each time a prompt is responded to, the capacitive sensor stores the information. The information can then be used to perform pattern matching and to see trends that clinicians may not be aware of. This information can be used to predict future action or for retrospective understanding.

Sensors	Prompts for action
Pedometers are used to monitor movement like walking or running.	There is ample evidence that early walking after surgery is beneficial for patient care. Pedometers can be used to encourage patients to walk after surgery.[148] Clinicians can receive prompts when those under their care need to be encouraged to walk more or even to praise those that have achieved the exercise goals.
Barcode and QR code sensors measure reflected light to create an electrical image to represent the barcode. This is converted to a digital signal to read the barcode or QR code.	If an item is not on the shelf, scanning the barcode or QR code can trigger a search function to locate the nearest item in the vicinity. In hospitals, indoor location services can provide information.
Microphones and image sensors record sound and images in digital format.	Benedict Evans says that machine learning has opened up new ways for computers to analyse audio and image data. Computers could not really read audio, images or video before and now, increasingly, this has become possible. This means that image sensors and microphones become input devices that generate machine-readable data.[149]

Machine Learning

Benedict Evans, a well-known consultant and mobile analysist, provides us with a useful way to view machine learning.[150] There's much hype about machine learning and artificial intelligence, and we know in some vague sense that it's a big thing. At some level, we understand that it's about pattern matching and data. But there's also the sense that it is some form of superhuman intelligence that will solve any problem. The truth is that machine learning is just a step-change in automating very specific tasks.

A useful example might be a washing machine. Washing machines automate the washing of clothes. They're not intelligent. They don't know what water or clothes are. Most importantly, they're not general purpose machines. Even in the narrow domain of washing, they cannot be used for washing dishes.

Replacing Experts

There's some sense that with each wave of automation, we'll replace experts. But this simply isn't true. With the debut of Excel, it didn't replace accountants, it just provided another tool to work with. With the introduction of Photoshop, it didn't replace graphic designers, it only made them more productive. This is the same with machine learning – it will make jobs easier to do and help us see connections we didn't see before. It will give us another tool to work with at scale.

A more nuanced way of looking at machine learning is perhaps that will be involved in:

- automation
- enabling technology
- relational databases.

Why Relational Databases?

Benedict Evans explains that databases were initially record-keeping systems. When they morphed into relational databases, they gave us the first business intelligence tool.[151] With relational databases, we could use SQL (the programming language used by computer administrators) to question the database about things that were difficult to know before, and receive answers with ease. For hospitals, it might be 'Which of our physicians use coronary stents and which brand do they prefer?'

These questions were not easy to obtain answers to before. Now, with machine generated information stored in relational databases, we could ask questions so that we could provide context-sensitive prompts. In a later article, Benedict Evans explores the role of machine learning in leveraging human capability.[152]

Human Leverage

Benedict Evans points out that the paradox of today's internet platforms is that they are vastly automated and have no human control or interaction over what any given person sees, and yet they are also totally dependent on human behaviour.[153] What they're really doing is observing, extracting and inferring things from what hundreds of millions of people do.

Too much data produces overload and degrades the value of the data itself. In other words, the challenge for internet platforms is how to add people at the right point of leverage to curate information. Evans also asks with machine learning how many people do we actually need to do this and do these people actually need to be on your platform.

Companies with Lots of Data Will Get Stronger

In another article, Evans[154] points out that there is a general misconception about data and machine learning. Many people believe that companies that have a lot of data will be able to command a greater market share in every market sector.

But more data only provides strength in narrow niche markets because machine learning can only be used to perform single or specific tasks. For instance, a computer that can play chess can only perform that single task. It cannot play any other board games with the chess data it has. Hence, a company that has a lot of chess data can only compete in the online chess game market – it cannot compete with companies that sell online checkers. In other words, machine learning cannot replicate the wide spectrum of capabilities that humans have. Machine learning is only another tool to be used.

Data Specificity

Although we need a lot of data for machine learning, the data use is specific to the problem to be solved. GE has a lot of telemetry data from gas turbines, Google has a lot of search data, and Amex has a lot of credit fraud data. But you can't use turbine data to find fraudulent transactions, just as you cannot use web searches to predict gas turbine failures. So whilst machine learning is a generalisable technology that can be used for many different kinds of applications, each application that is built can only be used to do one thing. This is similar to the washing machine example cited.

As I see it, hospitals are local entities. The datasets that each hospital needs for operational efficiency are specific to each hospital. Some data, such as data stored in country-wide registries will have use cases across all hospitals; however, this is beyond the scope of this book.

Motivated by Prompts

With information stored in relational databases, context-aware apps can learn exactly what a clinician needs in a specific situation and prompt them without compromising patient care. Context-aware devices are not new in hospitals. Hospitals already use context-aware devices such as intravenous medicine and fluid giving-sets, blood oximeters, heart-rate monitors and various imaging systems. These devices are focused on patient care, as it ought to be.

For the internal hospital supply chain, the benefit of receiving contextual-prompts on smartphones and other devices is a safety factor. For example, when the sensors pick up the information seamlessly in the environment, in which the clinician is attending to the patient, this information is communicated to their work group seamlessly, by recording the work performed. The information also highlights successful practices and processes.

Contextualising Materials

In hospitals, materials are used throughout the day. These materials are in constant flow with patient care. Finding materials and moveable assets is difficult. The task can be simplified by digitising materials. By doing this, nurses and clinicians will be able to touch the screens on their mobile devices to know what's available and locate the relevant materials they need.

By providing sensors in materials, computers can automatically keep track of constantly changing data. This can be done with materials by attaching RFID tags to packaging, then when information is picked up by sensors, everything becomes automated, that is, there's no need for people to order, receive, record usage, reorder, and even pay for materials.

With the use of smartphones, sensors and digitisation of materials, the hidden costs of materials management become easy to see and this can be incredibly valuable. Materials management has an important role to play in influencing both clinical and financial outcomes.[155] Financial considerations may not be the first concern for many doctors and nurses[156] in hospitals, but the business reality is, 'If no margin, then no mission'.[157]

Hospitals need greater transparency in healthcare costs. This is one of the few industries where costs are not visible.

Summary

- Putting contextual prompts in the way of motivated people can prove more successful in achieving outcomes than the use of education programmes, awareness campaigns, policy and procedures or even resorting to legislation.

- At present, machine learning ought to be seen as a step-change in hospitals.

- Contextual-prompts could influence and motivate clinicians to perform simple repetitious tasks consistently. Various prompts could influence clinicians to greater effort in their roles. Digitising materials with the use of sensors, computers and smartphones exposes hidden costs and inefficiencies that can be addressed.

7

—

Overcoming Hospital Challenges

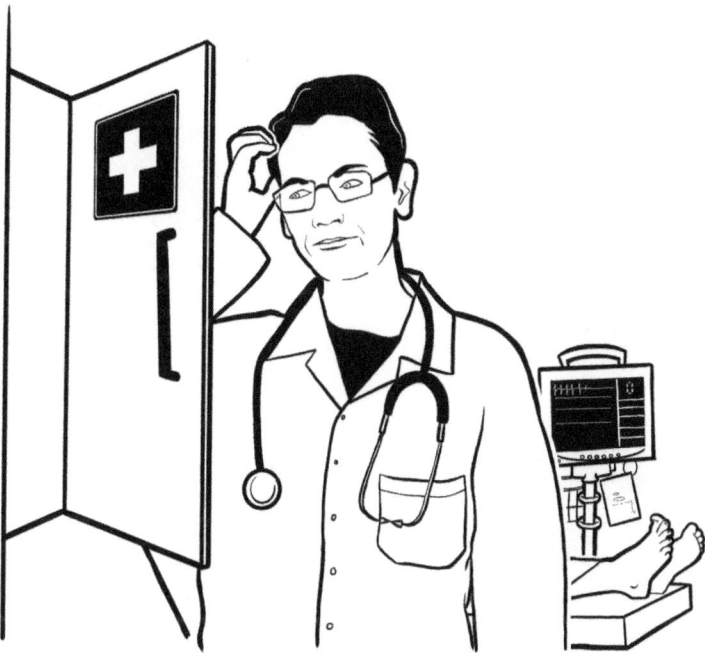

The major theme of this book is that technology has the potential to do things that nothing else can do. In terms of hospital workarounds, technology has the potential to succeed even where decades of education programs, awareness campaigns, product innovation and even legislation has failed. It has the potential to resolve hospital workarounds to keep patients safe from adverse events. However, to do this, technology must be applied using behaviour design insights.

The second theme of this book is that the psychological and physical distance of the architects of work – the high-level decision-makers – from the working interface encourages them to cram too many things into the work flow. This forces clinicians to multi-task, causing distractions. John Glaser, at the ECRI Annual Conference in 2017, commented that the intent of work, the actual jobs to be done was often diluted by the number of good ideas that were incorporated into information technology projects.[158]

Each idea in itself was good, but when all the ideas were aggregated, they crippled a project. As a result, clinicians are asked to collect more data in a structured way than is relevant to the performance of the job. This poses a risk to proper patient care.

Because the people that design jobs are far removed from the people that actually perform the jobs, they can only imagine how the job should be done. However, the job designed can lack context if rearranged incorrectly. Job architects rearrange tasks that often force clinicians to perform tasks that are not immediately required. Hence, jobs can be intentionally designed to gather information not actually required by the task at hand. The information is gathered because it could be used in different parts of the organisation. Unnecessary information gathering can cause an accumulation of errors.

The third theme of this book is that computers with sensors could close the gap between jobs as imagined and jobs as performed by providing shorter feedback loops to avoid the accumulation of errors.

The final theme of the book is that computers with sensors could sense the environment around them and automatically generate relevant information from the context that they are being used in. Computer-generated information can form the basis for data input rather than have people input data for machine analysis. In hospitals, context-awareness can be provided by digitising materials by using UHF-RFID labels.

These issues were corroborated by many speakers at the ECRI Institute's 2017 Annual Conference on 'Workflow, Workarounds, and Overworked Health Systems: Innovations and Challenges for Quality, Safety, and Technology'.

Lack of Time

It has been estimated that physicians and nurses spend twice as much time on documentation as on patient care. The time, or lack of it, was seen as one of the factors that impacted work burden, workflow and workarounds.

This book argues that with the use of context-aware computers in hospitals, this will be able to save clinicians and nurses time, and provide better safety for patients.

I will use the following format to demonstrate the application of these concepts to difficulties raised at the conference.

- Posing the problem
- Action
- Result

Problem 1 – The Inability to Track and Trace Items

The difficulty of tracking items appears to be a worldwide hospital phenomenon. The following is a case in point that most clinicians would relate to. The example is sited from the Ontario Hospital Association:[159]

> One of the most common surgical procedures, a straightforward laparoscopic cholecystectomy can be completed in less than an hour. But when the circulating nurse must leave the operating room (OR) in search of a new endo specimen retrieval bag because a labelling error had the cart loaded with the wrong size bag, things can change quickly. She searches the OR sterile core only to find its stock depleted.
>
> With the patient still on the operating table under aesthetic, calls must be made, other clinicians must be taken from their work to help and, eventually, the right size endo specimen retrieval bag found.
>
> Now the schedule has been shifted and the next surgery must begin late. What's more, staff members have lost confidence in the supply chain and some clinicians have already taken to stockpiling supplies to ward off another shortage.

Some surgical departments function in this manner because the time and effort it would take to overhaul an entire supply chain system is daunting.

I had earlier referred to the research conducted by Cohealo Inc. It is appropriate to repeat this here. The inability to track medical items and moveable assets results in a multimillion dollar black hole in hospital expenses. The outcome of such inability results in:

- a third or more surgeries at hospitals getting delayed or even postponed

- an additional $10 million capital expenditure per hospital

- nurses spending more than 20 minutes on each shift searching for items

- sixty percent of most inventory sitting idle in the hospital, in spite of being urgently needed.

Action

If hospitals use UHF-RFID labels for all the items delivered to the operating suite, they would be able to download an item checklist onto mobile RFID PDAs to do safety checks before the procedure begins. The scanner on the PDA would identify all the items available in the operating suite and produce an exception list of items missing.

In the example given above, the PDA would have identified that the endo specimen retrieval bag was missing. It would have highlighted that the wrong bag was in the operating suite, avoiding all the rework that had to be done to find the correct specimen bag.

If the device was connected to location services within the hospital, it would also identify where the nearest bag was located.

Result

In the case described, the following difficulties were identified and would have been resolved before the procedure began if a UHF-RFID infrastructure was used.

1. There was a labelling error. With UHF-RFID in use, the checks and balances with using a labelling process would have ruled out the possibility of such an error.

2. The OR sterile core stock was depleted. With UHF-RFID in use, automatic replenishment would eliminate this possibility. Information about stock on hand and status of replenishment would always be available on authorised devices.

3. The patient was on the operating table under aesthetic. With the UHF-RFID system in place, such eventualities are avoided. The missing item would have been flagged before the procedure began.

4. Other clinicians must be taken from their work to help. With UHF-RFID in use, such interruptions would have been avoided.

5. The schedule has been shifted and the next surgery must begin late. With UHF-RFID in use, the schedule is not disrupted due to material shortages.

6. Staff members have lost confidence in the supply chain and some clinicians have already taken to stockpiling supplies to ward off another shortage. With UHF-RFID in use, confidence in the supply chain function will be established and the need for individual stockpiles will be eliminated.

Problem 2 – Insulin Administration

Ronni P Solomon presented the following case during the ECRI 2017 Annual Conference.[160]

1. A patient needs insulin. The insulin is loaded into the automated dispensing cabinet.

2. The pharmacy generates a barcode on a separate paper to scan when administering the medication (because the medication is in a multi-dose vial). Scanning the barcode on the vial would constitute a multi-dose issue. The paper barcode allows a single dose issue.

3. On scanning the paper barcode, the nurse gets an error message – 'Patient has no order for the medication.' The incorrect barcode was generated by the pharmacy.

4. The nurse had no option but to override the error or scan the vial.

5. The protocol could not be followed.

Action

In the problem as presented, the process is extremely manual and had probably been designed in this way to force compliance for use of the automatic dispensing cabinet.

In hospitals where I have seen automatic dispensing cabinets used, the protocol is to dispense medication for one patient at a time. This is to ensure that the correct medication is dispensed for the right patient to avoid harm. Because dispensing units are situated in treatment rooms some distance from the patient's bedside, nurses tend to dispense medication sequentially for several patients at the same time. This saves time but poses the very risk that the design of work is trying to avoid.

Several alternatives offer themselves up for saving time and effort and for safety.

A secure mobile medication cart could be used, which could be wheeled to a given patient's bedside. As the carer approaches a resident, proximity sensors in their smart devices bring up the resident's relevant records, in this case, it would be their medication.

All that's now required is for the medication to be compared against the touchscreen checklist on the cart. Background algorithms take care of the recordkeeping and trigger associated synchronisation with other systems.

In the absence of mobile medication carts, the patient's bedside locker could be used. In this instance, the electronic medical chart on the nurse's mobile device becomes the touchscreen checklist.

Result

By using such a system, the protocol becomes part of the process. There is no difference between the job as imagined and the job as done. Staff at the Townsville Prescare Portea facility, where this particular example is currently taking place, say that the process halves the amount of time and effort that carers would otherwise take.

Multi-dose administration can be solved by using suitable algorithms.

Problems 3–5 were presented by Ellen S Deutsch at the ECRI 2017 Annual Conference. The issue raised was similar, though the workarounds were different.[161]

Problem 3 – Barcode Incomplete

1. The nurse was unable to successfully scan the barcode of the medication before administering the medicine to the patient because the barcode was incomplete.

2. The nurse rang the pharmacy and was instructed to:

    a. type the patient's name and medicinal record number

    b. document the medication confirmation manually.

Action

The patient received the medication.

Result

The underlying problem was not solved.

Problem 4 – Incorrect Barcode Used

1. On scanning the barcode, an error message was received, 'Medication invalid'.

2. The pharmacy determined that the medication was non-formulary (formularies lists insurance carriers' preferred drugs). The nurse was instructed to:

    a. override the error message and administer the medication

    b. report the event to the facilities' incident and serious reporting system.

Action

The patient received the medication and there was documentation to support investigation and mitigation.

Result

Documentation indicated that the formulary was updated.

Problem 5 – Barcode Unable to be Scanned

1. A high-risk medication was brought to a patient in respiratory isolation.

2. The nurse was unable to scan the barcode before medication was administered because the barcode was incomplete.

3. The medication was administered.

4. The nurse returned to where high-risk medications are held, to scan another undamaged barcode of the similar medicine for documentation purposes.

5. The scanner indicated that this was not the correct medication for the patient.

Action

The nurse's action bypassed a safety mechanism.

Result

Patient hazard.

Computers as Brains Without Senses

We can assume that in these examples the hospital staff had to input information using scanners, keyboards and printers.

This is, as Kevin Ashton says, 20th-century thinking and completely unnecessary.

Our smartphones and PDAs bear testament to the ease with which computers can be bundled with sensors to sense the environment around them and to contextually prompt users to take appropriate action. Similarly, as is being argued in this book, if clinicians used context-aware computers in their devices the information could be machine generated. As a result, process errors can be fed back immediately and resolved.

Summary

- Technology has the potential to resolve hospital workarounds and keep patients safe from adverse events.

- The psychological and physical distance from the working interface can be bridged so that high-level executives can structure work so that it is less prone to distractions from multi-tasking.

- Computers with sensors provide quicker feedback loops so that the job as imagined is more aligned to the work as performed. Computers with sensors could eliminate the need for clinicians to input information into databases, enabling them to focus on their patients and limit overwork.

8

—

Ten Hidden Hospital Hazards

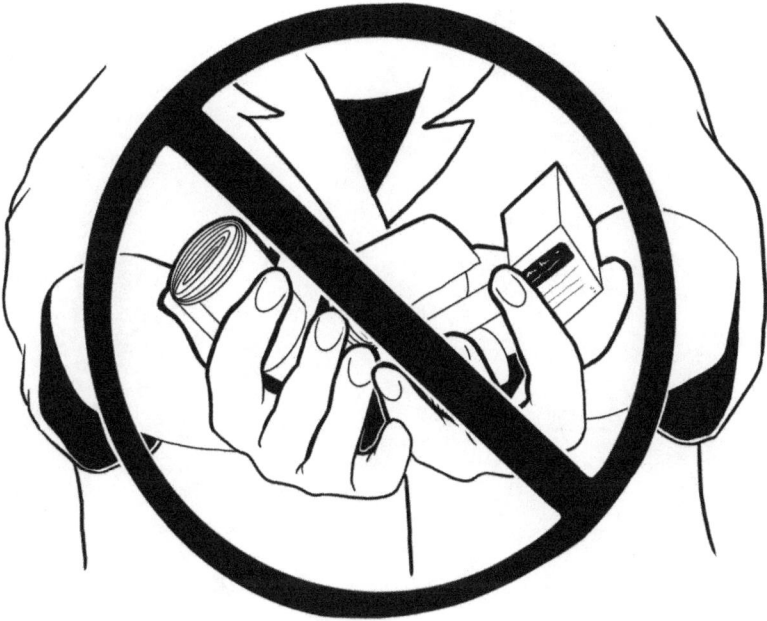

In this book, I have tried to make a case for using touch-to-know capability in hospitals. I believe, much like Clayton Christensen, Anita Tucker and others, that big problems can better be addressed by tackling small problems first.

Clayton Christensen's insight has been formed by studying disruption in business processes and in supply chains. Anita Tucker's insight was informed by observing the work in hospitals and seeing how small problems – because they're seen as too small to warrant attention – consume as much as a fifth of many nurses working days. [162]

Dave Brailsford, the British cycling coach, demonstrated that by making a 1% improvement in small things every day, this accumulated to a 37% improvement in efficiency. [163] He took the British Olympic Cycling Team in 2003 from mediocre performance to consistently win gold medals in most of their races.

I have identified ten hospital challenges that could all be solved using the touch-to-know capability. However, let me address briefly how the ten challenges can be tackled and addressed.

1 – Reduce Materials Costs

Hospitals aggregate costs, while clinicians are primarily concerned with patient care. By aggregating costs, hospitals are unable to match purchases with usage and accurately cost each procedure.

By using UHF-RFID technology, the hospital is able to create a closed loop. All items received are attached with RFID tags so that items can be traced and tracked through the hospital. The various stages of the item journey can be seen from receipt, storage, and eventual use.

The gap between purchase and usage is bridged and with the use of smart bins in each operating suite, procedure costing is obtained without any manual record-keeping.

Low cost imprest items could be tagged at the shelf-ready package level instead of the individual item level. When a shelf-ready package is opened and discarded, the antenna in the garbage area reads the tag and automatically depletes imprest stock, and reorders replenishment of the stock.

2 – Hiding Inventory

Because hospitals use thousands of items for patient care and these items are in constant movement with the patient flow, it is humanly impossible to track and trace these items. By using UHF-RFID, all items become visible. This eliminates the need to hide inventory. Private stashes of items become a thing of the past.

3 – No Time, No Space, No Materials

During the three decades that I have worked in hospitals, I've always heard clinicians and support services staff complain of the lack of time to complete all their tasks, the lack of space to store their materials and equipment, and the lack of materials themselves.

I believe that if we digitised information about hospital materials, assets and facilities, the limitations of time, space, and materials could be turned into assets. It is the inability to track and trace equipment and materials that prevent hospitals from using the business models adopted by Airbnb and companies similar to Uber. I will expand on this concept in the third book of this series.

4 – Keeping Patients Safe

I hope that I have shown how using context-aware computers with sensors will assist clinicians to avoid adverse events in hospitals. I believe that when machines gather information from the context of the work itself instead of getting busy clinicians to input information into computers, we will be able to provide them with context-aware prompts to keep patients safe in a complex and distracting workplace. The use of context-aware apps will be explored in more detail in book two of this series.

5 – Avoiding Human Error

Avoiding human error is a broader and more comprehensive aspect of patient safety. Whilst I have touched on this aspect in this book, the topic will be examined more fully in book two. It covers aspects beyond the internal hospital supply chain; however, the infrastructure adopted for digitising the internal hospital supply chain could be used to assist with the design of the work itself. This rapid feedback loop will assist in eliminating 'latent errors' as well as active errors due to distractions.

6 – Reducing Feedback Delay

As Benedict Evans says, one of the paradoxes of today's internet platforms is that they are vastly automated and have no human control or interaction over what any given person sees, and yet they are dependent on human behaviour.[164] This is because what they're doing is observing, extracting and inferring things from what hundreds of millions of people are doing.

The problem with generating such vast amounts of data is that the value of data degrades. If hospitals use the same data generation model, the amount of data generated is limited and context sensitive. It becomes an asset rather than a limitation.

Although the feedback loop has its uses for patient safety and for the prevention of human error, it must be seen as a tool in itself. This will be explored more fully in book two of the series.

7 – Avoiding Hospital Workarounds

Hospital workarounds are the symptoms of hidden root causes. It is my contention that by digitising the internal hospital supply chain, many of the root causes will be eliminated. If workarounds still exist, they will become more visible and become easier to solve.

8 – Physician Preference Items

Physician preference items are always a contentious issue, particularly around cost and standardisation. By digitising the internal hospital's supply chain, I believe hospitals will be able to transform their business model and, like Amazon, offer physicians the widest possible choice of items, delivered in time, at appropriate prices. This issue will be dealt with in more detail in book two of this series.

9 – Siloed Information

In hospitals, different departments have their own pool of information about products and this information is not suitably synchronised. As pointed out previously, data quality continuously deteriorates unless there is an ongoing systematic program to monitor data quality and prevent deterioration. By digitising information about materials and storing this information in the cloud, this will provide a single source of synchronised data. This could alleviate the communication problems that hospitals are currently facing.

10 – Improving Hospital Margins

Hospitals are facing a serious financial crisis because costs are increasing and reimbursement is falling. By digitising the internal supply chain, internal inefficiencies can be addressed. This in itself is a major step. With proper costings, claims, and other operational efficiencies I believe that hospitals can improve margins. By adopting a different business model, their margins can be increased further. Business models will form part of the third book in this series.

Let me end by paraphrasing Clayton Christensen: healthcare can be transformed by using technology to simplify tasks. They need a business model that they can use to take their simplified solution to market, and they need a supporting cast of suppliers and distributors that form part of a value network.[165]

This book deals with the technology that forms the basis for simplifying tasks for patient safety. Book two of the series will deal with procedure costing and other inventory management processes so that hospitals can offer physicians the items they wish to use. Book three of the series will deal with the business model and the supporting cast of suppliers and distributors.

Conclusion

Reflecting on
Hidden Hospital Problems

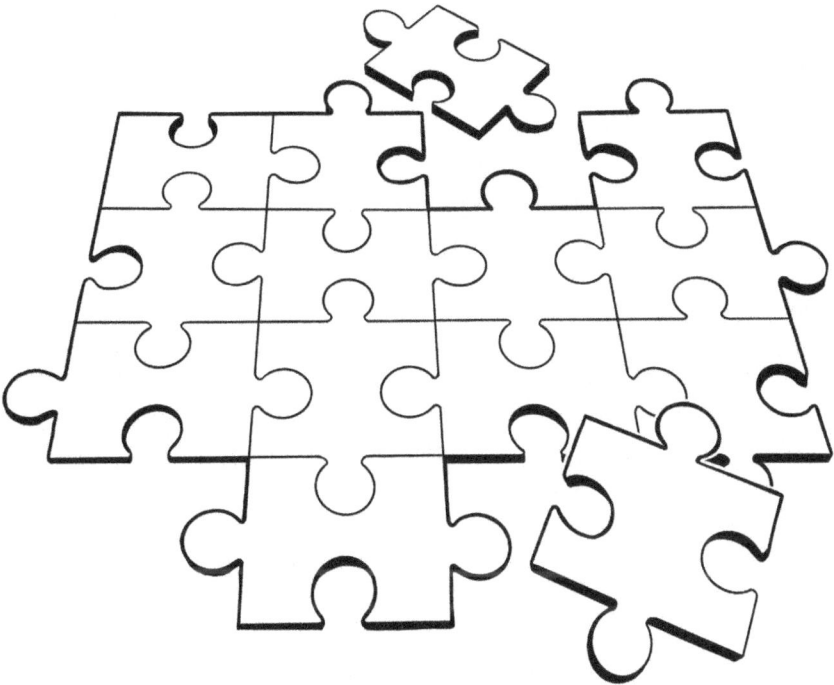

Reflecting on this journey, I can see that we were dealing with a wicked hospital problem. Charles Conn and Robert McLean identify *wicked problems* as those that defy an agreed problem definition and solution because they are intricately linked to complex human and technological systems.[166] These problems typically involve multiple causes, major value disagreements, complex interlinked systems, unintended consequences and seem to require substantial behaviour change.

Four aspects of the hospital problem, in keeping with Conn and McLean's views, are as follows:

The Problem Changes Shape as a Result of an Intervention

In Chapter 7 we see an example of this. John Glaser pointed out that the actual jobs done by physicians were diluted by the number of good ideas that get incorporated into information technology projects.[167] Each idea in itself was a good idea, but when all the ideas were aggregated, they crippled the project. As a result, clinicians were asked to collect more data in a structured way than was relevant to the performance of their jobs. This poses a risk to proper patient care.

There Appears to be No Such Thing as a Single Right Answer

In some hospitals, budgets are seen as performance management tools. Individual managers 'live or die' by their budgets. In these hospitals, internal fighting between departments over limited recourses results in poor service.

For example, the Engineering Services Department holds the budget for preventative maintenance. Maintenance costs are passed onto the departments that use their services. Gradually, as user departments dispute maintenance costs, the Engineering Services Department has to correspondingly reduce services to avoid budget overruns. This has a net reduced value in all areas.

Budgets must reflect real needs and budget variances must be justified based on these needs. The reality is that little time is spent by decision-makers to grapple with such variances. There are arguments on both sides of the situation and so the issue needs to be based on the least-loss outcome.

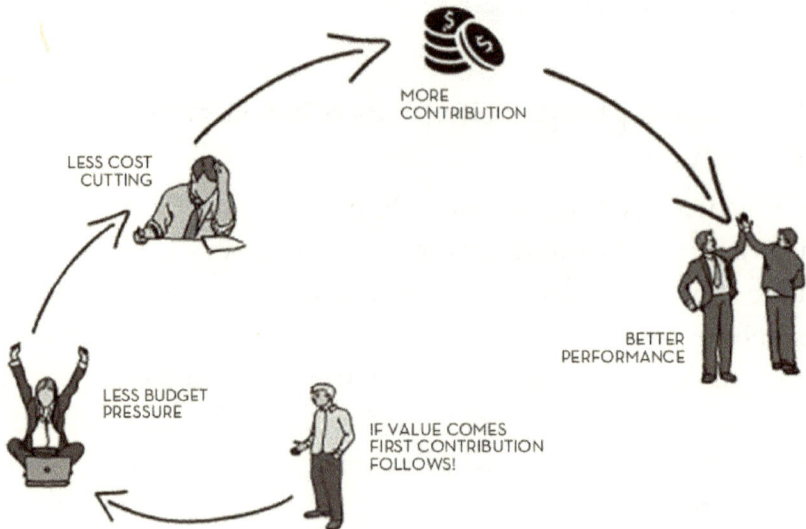

MORE CONTRIBUTION

LESS COST CUTTING

BETTER PERFORMANCE

LESS BUDGET PRESSURE

IF VALUE COMES FIRST CONTRIBUTION FOLLOWS!

I would argue, as Dave Gray does, that values come first, contribution follows. In budget-driven hospitals, employees that deliver value to internal customers without budgetary constraints will create a greater willingness for everybody to contribute more.

Differing Values Play an Important Role in Solving Problems

Early in 1988, when I first started working in the internal hospital supply chain in Australia, I was asked by our hospital executive to exclude Kaltostat from our procurement catalogue.

Kaltostat is an absorbent, haemostatic dressing, which forms a viscous gel on contact with bleeding wounds. It maintains its integrity when gelled, allowing one-piece removal with minimal pain to the patient.

At that time, excluding Kaltostat was an easy instruction to follow. Kaltostat was two hundred times more expensive than cotton gauze, the cheaper alternative. The issue with cotton gauze was that it often adhered to open wounds and was physically painful for the patient.

A short time after I removed Kaltostat from our catalogue, I was admitted to hospital for the removal of a nasal polyp. The physician who performed the procedure warned me that the removal of my dressing after the operation would be painful especially as the effect of the anaesthetic would have worn off.

When he did remove the dressing, I commented, 'That was easy!'

'Yes, that was the last of the Kaltostat I had. Some idiot in procurement has decided to stop purchasing this dressing.'

I have been uncomfortable with making decisions that go against physician preference items since then. I'm hoping that the solution I am now offering hospitals would be able to bring people with different value systems together to discuss all aspects of the value equation with hard data that's shared to support differing views.

The Real Problem Is Not Always the Presenting Problem

Charles Conn and Robert McLean observe that with wicked problems, the real problems are nested inside other, more apparent problems.[168] When I visited our operating suites in April 2011, I had visualised the problem as providing clinicians with an easier way to list the items they used in a procedure. The problem turned out to be instead about reducing anxiety and using context-aware computers in hospitals instead.

Seven Steps

In hindsight, it would appear that I have used Charles Conn and Robert McLean's seven steps out of consciousness. Let me outline how the seven steps informed my thoughts and actions in formulating my touch-to-know approach.

1. Define the problem

When I first embarked on this journey, I thought I had a clear idea of what the problem was. Nurses weren't accurately listing the items that they used during their procedures. However, when I visited the operating suite to demonstrate how nurses could do their jobs to accurately list the items they used during a procedure, I realised the problem was more complex than I had first visualised.

The problem was, in fact, of poor work design. By insisting that nurses listed the items that they used during a procedure, we were distracting them from their primary task of patient care. We were encouraging errors to be made and detracting from providing safe care.

I eventually defined the problem as 'How could the use of materials contribute to safe patient care?' The use of technology to gather information without manual intervention then became an enabling issue in the service of patient safety and did not detract from patient care.

2. Disaggregating the issues

Once the problem was defined, I broke it down into its component parts. I gradually came to realise that the many workarounds that I encountered with the supply of materials were in fact opportunities to improve the process.

For example, hiding inventory is an open secret in hospitals. However, I've always viewed it a poor work practice on the part of nurses rather than a problem to be addressed as a supply chain function. My function, as I saw it, was with the procurement and delivery of items to the wards and operating suites.

Once the items were delivered, the accounting and safekeeping of the items were the responsibility of the clinicians using the products. This boundary issue eventually became 'How do I help nurses track and trace the thousands of items they use on a daily basis?'

This was a significant issue because it is humanly impossible to keep track of the many items in constant circulation in a hospital.

3 Prioritising the issues

Focusing on hiding eventually helped to unravel the problem of safety with materials in its entirety. The other issues in relation to tagging the product, the process flow and the use of enabling technology were dovetailed into the critical path for rolling out the solution.

4 Committing to a work plan

Once I determined what the component parts and the priorities for each part of the problem it was easy to link each part to a plan. Rather than involve internal stakeholders at the hospital, I decided to use external consultants and application designers to assist me. In hindsight, this was a big mistake. While it was easier to get the work done, buy-in required for the full rollout of the solution was lacking. As Dr Simon Woods, Medical Director for Cabrini Health at the time, said, 'There was no issue with the solution; the issue was that I had not obtained buy-in from the people impacted the most.'

5. Analysing information, hard data and qualitative information

It was fortunate that I and some of the members of my supply chain team had access to the hospital ERP database. By using SQL, we were able to obtain and analyse the effectiveness of our implementation. Qualitative data was obtained from continued daily discussions with the nursing staff on the wards and in the operating suite.

6. Synthesising our thinking and our feelings

Unfortunately, as Conn and McLean say: problem-solving doesn't stop at the point of reaching conclusions from individual analyses. Findings need to be constructed into a logical structure, validated and then used to convince others that the solution is useful. Great team processes are important. As I pointed out earlier, this was my mistake. I'd decided that forming a team outside my own department would delay the process. As a result, I had a workable solution but had not gained management sanction to implement the solution fully.

7. Preparing powerful communication

The final step was to develop a storyline from the conclusions that link back to the problem statement and the issues that were defined. The story would then lead to action steps or pose a series of further questions that motivates action depending on the audience and receptivity. I had, in my haste, been unable to develop the story.

I'm now doing so with the publication of this book. I hope that I will now reach a wider and more receptive hospital audience that will identify with and implement the 'touch-to-know' solution in their hospitals. Introducing context-aware computers into hospitals is only the beginning. If this solution has to gain traction in hospitals, Conn & McLean's seven steps must now be used consciously with intent.

Or as T S Eliot says, 'What we call the beginning is often the end. And to make an end is to make a beginning. The end is where we start from.'

Acknowledgements

I have benefited enormously from working with colleagues in solving problems over the past 50 years in many different industries. During the last 30 years, I was fortunate enough to work in hospitals. Over the years, I have worked with many creative people and apologise that I cannot mention all of them.

Let me begin by thanking Geoff Fazakerley with whom I've worked with for the past 19 years at Cabrini in what I consider was the most meaningful working period of my life. It was Geoff who gave me the opportunity to work with computers and to automate business processes to assist clinicians to provide better care.

My thanks to Dr Michael Walsh, CEO of Cabrini Health and Dr Simon Woods, previously Medical Director for Cabrini Health for giving me access to the operating suites and freeing up time for their clinicians to meet with me. I thank Chintan Shah and Chaminda Moragoda my work colleagues for the many hours they put in to assist me with the many practical problems I faced with tracking and tracing inventory.

I thank Craig Potter and David Walmsley, two JDE application consultants for their patience in teaching me about relational databases. They taught me how to build databases and how to use SQL to extract information that was distributed across several tables.

I want to thank Bev, my wife, for making this book possible. Her constant pruning of technical jargon makes this a more readable book. Bev helped me bridge the gap between my thinking and my expression and by insisting that I explain myself more clearly.

I pay homage to the many authors who have informed my work. Too many to name individually. However, I must mention Chris Anderson, who opened my eyes to the demise of over-standardisation and the possibilities of endless choice.

I have gained tremendous insight from Joe Pine and the work of his co-authors. They have influenced my thinking over the years. Don Norman and James Reason alerted me to the ways in which system architects inadvertently design latent errors into complex systems and how to avoid such mistakes.

Kevin Ashton helped me see the role that context-aware computers could play in freeing up time for clinicians in hospitals. B J Fogg helped me understand how placing prompts in the way of motivated people could ensure that behaviours are successfully completed.

I thank James Currier and Ben Thompson for the insight they provided on network effects and aggregation theory. I'd like to thank Benedict Evans for his weekly newsletter that kept me abreast of what was happening in the world of technology. Charles Conn and Robert McLean helped me see that good problem-solving without the involvement of key stakeholders were bound to fail.

I am grateful to Saul Resnick, CEO Australia, DHL Supply Chain, Michael Gardner, Vice President Life Sciences DHL Australia, Mark Holden, Commercial Manager, DHL Supply

Chain Australia, Chris Sheehan, GM Operations, DHL Supply Chain and John Ioannou, Business Manager, DHL Supply Chain Australia for their tutelage into the intricacies of large scale warehousing and distribution.

Finally, I must thank Blaise van Hecke and Scott Vandervalk from Busybird Publishing for their advice and the many hours they spent in getting this book published.

Endnotes

1. David Price (2013), *Open: How we'll work, live and learn in the future*, Crux Publishing, Great Britain.

2. Charles Conn and Robert McLean (2018), *Bulletproof Problem Solving: The One Skill that Changes Everything*, John Wiley & Sons, Inc., Hoboken, New Jersey.

3. Steven Johnson (2013), 'Recognising the true potential of technology to change behaviour', https://www.theguardian.com/sustainable-business/behavioural-insights/true-potential-technology-change-behaviour.

4. Jonathan S Skinner (2013), 'The costly paradox of health-care technology', https://www.technologyreview.com/s/518876/the-costly-paradox-of-health-care-technology.

5. Dave Gray and Thomas Vander Wal (2014), *The Connected Company*, O'Reilly Media, 1005 Gravenstein Highway North, Sebastopol, CA 9542 and ECRI Institute's 2017 Annual Conference: Workflow, Workarounds, and Overworked Health Systems: Innovations and Challenges for Quality, Safety, and Technology, https://www.youtube.com/playlist?list=PLEvm6gjNpayM15XmCXOCase_gEiUFiSMm.

6. (ibid) James Reason (2008), *The Human Contribution: Unsafe Acts, Accidents and Heroic Recoveries*, CRC Press.

7. James Reason (2009), *Human Error*, Cambridge University Press.

8. James Reason (2008), *The Human Contribution: Unsafe Acts, Accidents and Heroic Recoveries*, CRC Press

9. See footage from ECRI Institute's 2017 Annual Conference.

10. Op cite Dave Gray and Thomas Vander Wal (2014).

11. David J Hillis, David AK Watters, Lawrie Malisano, Nick Bailey and David Rankin (2017), 'Variation in the costs of surgery: Seeking value', https://www.mja.com.au/journal/2017/206/4/variation-costs-surgery-seeking-value.

12. 'Learning the right lessons from past accidents', in James Reason (1990), *Human Error*, Cambridge University Press, 32 Avenue of the Americas, New York, NY10013-2473, USA.

13. Thomas R Krause, PhD., and John H Hindley, MD (2009), *Taking the Lead in Patient Safety: How Healthcare Leaders Influence Behaviour and Create Culture*, John Wiley & Sons, Inc., Hoboken, New York.

14. 'Defining and classifying error', in James Reason (1990), *Human Error*, Cambridge University Press, 32 Avenue of the Americas, New York, NY10013-2473, USA.
'Intended actions and mistakes', in James Reason (2008), *The Human Contribution: Unsafe Acts, Accidents and Heroic Recoveries*, CRC Press, Taylor Francis Group, Boca Raton, London, New York.
'Two types of errors: slips and mistakes', in Don Norman (2013), *The Design of Everyday Things: Revised and Expanded Edition*, Basic Books, New York.

15. Kevin Ashton (2015), *How to Fly a Horse: The Secret History of Invention*, William Heinemann, 20 Vauxhall Bridge Road, London SW1V 2SA.

16. Cynthia Barton Rabe (2006), *The Innovation Killer: How What We Know Limits What We Can Imagine And What Smart Companies Are Doing About It*, American Management Association, New York.

17. James Reason (2008), *The Human Contribution: Unsafe Acts, Accidents and Heroic Recoveries*, CRC Press, Taylor Francis Group, Boca Raton, London, New York.
Thomas R. Krause, Ph.D., and John H. Hindley, M.D. (2009), *Taking the Lead in Patient Safety: How Healthcare Leaders Influence Behaviour and Create Culture*, John Wiley & Sons, Inc., Hoboken, New York
James Reason (1990), *Human Error*, Cambridge University Press, 32 Avenue of the Americas, New York, NY10013-2473, USA.

18. Don Norman (2013), *The Design of Everyday Things: Revised and Expanded Edition*, Basic Books, New York

19. Op cite – Don Norman (2013), *The Design of Everyday Things: Revised and Expanded Edition*, Basic Books, New York.

20. Clayton M Christensen, Jerome H. Grossman, MD, and Jason Hwang, MD, (2009), *The Innovator's Prescription: A Disruptive Solution for Health Care*, McGraw Hill Companies, Inc. New York.

21. James Reason (1990), *Human Error*, Cambridge University Press, 32 Avenue of the Americas, New York, NY10013-2473, USA.

22. Kevin Ashton (2015), *How to Fly a Horse: The Secret History of Invention*, William Heinemann, 20 Vauxhall Bridge Road, London SW1V 2SA.

23. Benedict Evans (2016), 'Mobile ate the world', Andreessen Horowitz, https://www.slideshare.net/a16z/mobile-is-eating-the-world-2016.

24. Enu Waktola (2015), 'RAIN Q&A with Kevin Ashton: RAIN and the Internet of Things', https://rainrfid.org/wp-content/uploads/2015/12/Kevin-Ashton.pdf.

25. Calum McClelland (2017), https://www.leverege.com/blogpost/what-is-iot-simple-explanation.

26. James Manyika, Michael Chui, Peter Bisson, Jonathan Woetzel, Richard Dobbs, Jacques Bughin, and Dan Aharon (2015), 'The Internet of Things: Mapping the Value Beyond the Hype', McKinsey & Company, https://www.mckinsey.com/business-functions/digital-mckinsey/our-insights/the-internet-of-things-the-value-of-digitizing-the-physical-world.

27. Enu Waktola (2015), 'RAIN Q&A with Kevin Ashton: RAIN and the Internet of Things', https://rainrfid.org/wp-content/uploads/2015/12/Kevin-Ashton.pdf.

28. Clayton M Christensen, Ridgway Harken Hall, Karen Dillion, and David S Duncan, (2016), *Competing Against Luck: The Story of Innovation and Customer Choice*, Harper Collins Publishers Australia Pty. Ltd, Level 13, 201 Elizabeth Street, Sydney, NSW 2000, Australia.

29. Fred Kimball (2015), *Is Your Inventory Accuracy Really As Good As Your Auditor's Report,* Distribution Design Inc., https://distributiondesign.com.

30. David J Hillis, David AK Watters, Lawrie Malisano, Nick Bailey and David Rankin (2017), 'Variation in the costs of surgery: seeking value', https://www.mja.com.au/journal/2017/206/4/variation-costs-surgery-seeking-value.

31. *Anita Tucker in* Frances Frei, Anne Morriss (2012), *Uncommon Service: How to win by putting customers at the core of your business,* Harvard Business Review Press.

32. James Reason (2008), *The Human Contribution: Unsafe Acts, Accidents and Heroic Recoveries*, CRC Press, Taylor Francis Group, Boca Raton, London, New York.

33. Australian Hospital Patient Costing Standards (2018), https://www.ihpa.gov.au/publications/australian-hospital-patient-costing-standards-version-40.

34. Isabel Menzies Lyth (1960), http://moderntimesworkplace.com/archives/ericsess/sessvol1/Lythp439.opd.pdf.

35. Cohealo (2018), 'Taking Aim At A Multi-Million Dollar Blind Spot: How Underutilized Medical Equipment is Shrinking Hospital Margins'.

36. Len Kennedy (2016), 'How No-Time, No-Space, No-Materials Disrupts Hospital Supply Chains', National Supply Chain Conference, Sydney.

37. Sangeet Paul Choudary (2015), *Platform Scale: How An Emerging Business Model Helps Startups Build Large Empires with Minimum Investment*, Platform Thinking Labs Pte. Ltd.

Geoffrey G Parker, Marshall W Van Alstyne, and Sangeet Paul Choudary (2016), *Platform Revolution: How Networked Markets are Transforming the Economy and How to Make Them Work for You*, W.W. Norton & Company, Inc., 500 Fifth Avenue, New York, NY 10110.

Alex Moazed and Nicholas L Johnson (2016), *Modern Monopolies: What It Takes to Dominate the 21st Century Economy*, St. Martin's Press, New York.

38. This would be similar to what Amazon is endeavouring to do. See Brad Scott (2013), *The Everything Store*, Transworld Publishers, 61-63 Uxbridge Road, London W 5 5SA.

39. Australian Government, Australian Institute of Health and Welfare, Australia's Hospitals, 2013.

40. Andrew Barton-Jones (2018): 'Digital hospitals: The verdict so far…' https://stories.uq.edu.au/momentum-magazine/2018/future-of-health/index.html.

41. Kevin Ashton (2015), *How to Fly a Horse: The Secret History of Invention*, William Heinemann, 20 Vauxhall Bridge Road, London SW1V 2SA.

42. The Institute of Medicine (2000). *To Err Is Human: Building a Safer Health System*. Washington, DC: The National Academies Press. doi:10.17226/9728. ISBN 978-0-309-26174-6 (in https://en.wikipedia.org/wiki/Medical_error#cite_note-toerr-9).

43. Clinicians need 'error wisdom' at their fingertips, in James Reason (2008), *The Human Contribution: Unsafe Acts, Accidents and Heroic Recoveries*, CRC Press, Taylor Francis Group, Boca Raton, London, New York.

44. B J Fogg (2003), *Persuasive Technology: Using Computers to Change What We Think and Do*, Morgan Kaufmann Publishers, 340 Pine Street, Sixth Floor, San Francisco, CA 94104-3205.

45. Nir Eyal (2014), *Hooked: How to Build Habit-Forming Products*, Penguin Books Ltd., 80 Strand, London WC2R 0RL, England.

46. James Reason (2008), *The Human Contribution: Unsafe Acts, Accidents and Heroic Recoveries*, CRC Press, Taylor Francis Group, Boca Raton, London, New York.

Charles Haddon-Cave QC (2006), 'The Nimrod Review: An independent review into the broader issues surrounding the loss of the RAF Nimrod MR2 Aircraft XV230 in Afghanistan in 2006', HC1025 London: Stationery Office.

Thomas R Krause, PhD., and John H Hindley, MD (2009), *Taking the Lead in Patient Safety: How Healthcare Leaders Influence Behaviour and Create Culture*, John Wiley & Sons, Inc., Hoboken, New York.

47. The 'five-rules-in-use' in (Clayton M Christensen, Jerome H Grossman, MD, and Jason Hwang, MD, (2009), 'The Innovator's Prescription: A Disruptive Solution for Health Care', McGraw Hill Companies, Inc. New York.

48. James Clear (2018), *Atomic Habits: An Easy and Proven Way to Build Good Habits and Break Bad Ones*, Random House Business Books, The Penguin Random House Group Limited, 20 Vauxhall Bridge Road, London, SW1V 2SA.

49. James Reason (2008), *The Human Contribution: Unsafe Acts, Accidents and Heroic Recoveries*, CRC Press, Taylor Francis Group, Boca Raton, London, New York. James Reason (1990), *Human Error*, Cambridge University Press, 32 Avenue of the Americas, New York, NY10013-2473, USA.

50. Anita Tucker in Frances Frei, Anne Morriss (2012), *Uncommon Service: How to win by putting customers at the core of your business,* Harvard Business Review Press.

51. Simon Woods (2015), 'Challenges and Opportunities in Procurement: A Private Hospital Perspective', The National Procurement Conference, Menzies Hotel, Sydney.

52. Adi Ignatius, 'Jeff Bezos on Leading for the Long-Term at Amazon,' *HBR IdeaCast* (blog), *Harvard Business Review,* January 3, http://blogs.hbr.org/ideacast/2013/01/jeff-bezos-onleading-for-the.html. In Brad Stone (2013), 'The Everything Store: Jeff Bezos and the Age of Amazon', Transworld Publishers, 61-63 Uxbridge Road, London W5 5SA.

53. Ontario Hospital Association, 'Optimizing Your Perioperative Supply Chain: A Guide to Improvement Projects'.

54. Arkady Maydanchik (2007), *Data Quality for Practitioners Series: Data Quality Assessment*, Technics Publications, LLC Bradley Beach, NJ07720 USA.

55. Ian Robertson (2011), *Improving Supply Chains Using RFID & Standards*, Supply Chain RFID Consulting, LLC., 7607 Langley Road, Spring, Texas 77389-5051 USA.

56. Norman Swan (2015): http://www.abc.net.au/radionational/programs/bigideas/can-australian-health-care-be-saved/6969426.

57. Rob O'Byrne (2016), https://www.logisticsbureau.com/nursing-hospital-and-healthcare-supply-into-a-new-age.

58. To understand this approach we need to examine the platform business model that has been extensively examined by several business authors. However, in hospitals this approach can only be undertaken if all hospital materials and moveable assets are digitised.

59. B Joseph Pine II, Kim C Korn (2011), *Infinite Possibility: Creating Customer Value on the Digital Frontier*, Berrett-Koehler Publishers, Inc., San Francisco, California 94104-291.

60. Kevin Ashton (2015), *How to Fly a Horse: The Secret History of Invention*, William Heinemann, 20 Vauxhall Bridge Road, London SW1V 2SA.

61. Josh Fruhlinger and Thomas Waligum (2017), '15 Famous ERP Disasters, Dustups, and Disappointments',

62. Oliver Champion-Awwad, Alexander Hayton, Leila Smith, and Mark Vuaran (2014), 'The National Programme for IT in the NHS: A Case History', https://www.cl.cam.ac.uk/~rja14/Papers/npfit-mpp-2014-case-history.pdf.

63. Jim Birch and Tim Kelsey (2016), 'Your Health. Your Say – Shaping the future of health and care together: A consultation with the Australian community to co-produce the National Digital Health Strategy', A Discussion Paper, https://www.digitalhealth.gov.au/about-the-agency/australian-digital-health-agency-board/board-papers/7.2%20-%20Update%20on%20National%20Strategy%20Engagement%20Project-%20Attachment%20A.pdf.

64. Stefan Biesdorf and Florian Niedermann (July 2014), 'Healthcare's Digital Future', https://www.mckinsey.com/industries/healthcare-systems-and-services/our-insights/healthcares-digital-future.

65. Kevin Ashton (2015), *How to Fly a Horse: The Secret History of Invention*, William Heinemann, 20 Vauxhall Bridge Road, London SW1V 2SA.

66. Andrew Barton-Jones (2018): 'Digital Hospitals: The Verdict so far…' https://stories.uq.edu.au/momentum-magazine/2018/future-of-health/index.html.

67. Stefan Biesdorf and Florian Niedermann (July 2014), 'Healthcare's Digital Future', https://www.mckinsey.com/industries/healthcare-systems-and-services/our-insights/healthcares-digital-future.

68. Oliver Champion-Awwad, Alexander Hayton, Leila Smith, and Mark Vuaran (2014), 'The National Programme for IT in the NHS: A Case History', https://www.cl.cam.ac.uk/~rja14/Papers/npfit-mpp-2014-case-history.pdf.

69. Today many such services can also be delivered by voice.

70. Dr Nicole Gillespie, 'Rolling out the healthcare revolution', https://www.business.uq.edu.au/momentum/rolling-out-healthcare-revolution.

71. Steven Johnson (2013), 'Recognising the true potential of technology to change behaviour', https://www.theguardian.com/sustainable-business/behavioural-insights/true-potential-technology-change-behaviour.

72. Clayton M. Christensen, Jerome H. Grossman, M.D., and Jason Hwang, M.D., (2009), *The Innovator's Prescription: A Disruptive Solution for Health Care*, McGraw Hill Companies, Inc. New York.

73. Jonathan Bush and Stephen Baker (2014), *Where Does It Hurt? An Entrepreneur's Guide to Fixing Health-Care*, (Copyright Athena Health. Inc., Penguin Group (USA) LLC, 375 Hudson Street, New York 10014.

74. https://www.aihw.gov.au/reports/australias-health/australias-health-2018/contents/indicators-of-australias-health/potentially-avoidable-deaths.

75. https://www.digitalhealth.gov.au/news-and-events/news/tim-kelsey-digital-opportunities-in-health-services.

76. Atul Gawande (2002, 2003, 2010), *Complications: A Surgeon's Notes on an Imperfect Science*, Profile Books, 3A Exmouth House, Pine Street, Exmouth Market, London EC1R 0JH.

77. Dave Gray and Thomas Vander Wal (2014), *The Connected Company*, O'Reilly Media, 1005 Gravenstein Highway North, Sebastopol, CA 9542.

78. David J Hillis, David AK Watters, Lawrie Malisano, Nick Bailey and David Rankin (2017), 'Variation in the costs of surgery: seeking value', https://www.mja.com.au/journal/2017/206/4/variation-costs-surgery-seeking-value.

79. ECRI Institute's 2017 Annual Conference: Workflow, Workarounds, and Overworked Health Systems: Innovations and Challenges for Quality, Safety, and Technology, https://www.youtube.com/playlist?list=PLEvm6gjNpayM15XmCXOCase_gEiUFiSMm.

80. Session 4: When Workarounds Are the Norm in Clinical Care, ECRI Institute, https://www.youtube.com/watch?v=yQfZT2pdREM&t=271s.

81. Sangeet Paul Choudary (2015), *Platform Scale: How an emerging business model helps startups build large empires with minimum investment*, Platform Thinking Labs Pte. Ltd
Geoffrey G Parker, Marshall W. Van Alstyne, and Sangeet Paul Choudary (2016), 'Platform Revolution: How Networked Markets are Transforming the Economy and How to Make Them Work for You', W.W. Norton & Company, Inc., 500 Fifth Avenue, New York, NY 10110
Alex Moazed and Nicholas L. Johnson (2016), *Modern Monopolies: What It Takes to Dominate the 21st Century Economy*, St. Martin's Press, New York.

82. The hospital business model could be better understood and redesigned if necessary using Alexander Osterwalder and Yves Pigneur (2010), *Business Model Generation: A Handbook for Visionaries, Game Changers, and Challengers*, John Wiley & Sons Inc., Hoboken, New Jersey.

83. Atul Gawande (2002, 2003, 2010), *Complications: A Surgeon's Notes on an Imperfect Science*, Profile Books, 3A Exmouth House, Pine Street, Exmouth Market, London EC1R 0JH.

84. Ian Robertson (2011), *Improving Supply Chains Using RFID & Standards*, Supply Chain RFID Consulting, LLC., 7607 Langley Road, Spring, Texas 77389-5051 USA.

85. Fred Kimball (2015), *Is Your Inventory Accuracy Really As Good As Your Auditor's Report*, Distribution Design Inc., https://distributiondesign.com.

86. James Reason (2008), *The Human Contribution: Unsafe Acts, Accidents and Heroic Recoveries*, CRC Press, Taylor Francis Group, Boca Raton, London, New York.

87. Cynthia Barton Rabe (2006), *The Innovation Killer: How What We Know Limits What We Can Imagine And What Smart Companies Are Doing About It*, American Management Association, New York.

88. Calum McClelland (2017). https://www.leverege.com/blogpost/what-is-iot-simple-explanation.

89. Michael J McGrath and Cilodhana Ni Scanaill (2014), *Sensor Technologies: Healthcare, Wellness and Environmental Applications*, Apress Media

90. Calum McClelland (2017). https://www.leverege.com/blogpost/what-is-iot-simple-explanation.

Kevin Ashton (2015), *How to Fly a Horse: The Secret History of Invention*, William Heinemann, 20 Vauxhall Bridge Road, London SW1V 2SA.

91. Jeff Bezos (2003) 'The Electricity Metaphor', https://www.ted.com/talks/jeff_bezos_on_the_next_web_innovation?language=en.

92. Evan Andrews (2013), 'Who Invented the Internet?' https://www.history.com/news/who-invented-the-internet.

93. Jonathan Bush and Stephen Baker (2014), 'Where does it hurt? An Entrepreneur's Guide to Fixing Health-Care', (Copyright Athena Health. Inc., Penguin Group (USA) LLC, 375 Hudson Street, New York 10014.

94. Dave Gray and Thomas Vander Wal (2014), *The Connected Company*, O'Reilly Media, 1005 Gravenstein Highway North, Sebastopol, CA 9542.

95. Ian Robertson (2011), *Improving Supply Chains Using RFID & Standards*, Supply Chain RFID Consulting, LLC., 7607 Langley Road, Spring, Texas 77389-5051 USA.

96. Jonathan Bush and Stephen Baker (2014) op cit.

97. Fred Lee (2004), *If Disney Ran Your Hospital: The 9½ Things You Would Do Differently*, Second River Healthcare Press.

98. Martin Bowles (2015) The Secretary of the Federal Department of Health: http://www.abc.net.au/radionational/programs/bigideas/can-australian-health-care-be-saved/6969426.

99. Clayton M. Christensen, Jerome H. Grossman, M.D., and Jason Hwang, M.D., (2009), *The Innovator's Prescription: A Disruptive Solution for Health Care*, McGraw Hill Companies, Inc. New York.

100. Australian Government, Australian Institute of Health and Welfare, Australia's Hospitals 2013–14.

101. James Reason (2008), *The Human Contribution: Unsafe Acts, Accidents and Heroic Recoveries*, CRC Press, Taylor Francis Group, Boca Raton, London, New York.

102. Anand Swaminathan and Jürgen Meffert (2017), *Digital@Scale: How you can lead your business with Digital@Scale*, Copyright McKinsey & Company, John Wiley & Sons, Inc. Hoboken, New Jersey.

103. N R Krishnan and A. S. Kasthuri (2005), 'Iatrogenic Disorders', https://www.ncbi.nlm.nih.gov/pmc/articles/PMC4923397.

104. Anita Tucker (2013), 'An Obstacle to Patient Centred Care: Poor Supply Systems', HBR, https://hbr.org/2013/10/an-obstacle-to-patient-centered-care-poor-supply-systems.

105. Clayton M Christensen, Jerome H Grossman, MD, and Jason Hwang, MD, (2009), *The Innovator's Prescription: A Disruptive Solution for Health Care*, McGraw Hill Companies, Inc. New York.

106. Sangeet Paul Choudary (2015), *Platform Scale: How an emerging business model helps startups build large empires with minimum investment*, Platform Thinking Labs Pte. Ltd.
Geoffrey G Parker, Marshall W Van Alstyne, and Sangeet Paul Choudary (2016), *Platform Revolution: How Networked Markets are Transforming the Economy and How to Make Them Work for You*, W W Norton & Company, Inc., 500 Fifth Avenue, New York, NY 10110.
Alex Moazed and Nicholas L Johnson (2016), *Modern Monopolies: What It Takes to Dominate the 21st Century Economy*, St. Martin's Press, New York.

107. Writers about the platform business model refer to customers, buyers, and sellers as users as the roles can be interchangeable depending on the context of the transaction.

108. Clayton M Christensen, Jerome H Grossman, MD, and Jason Hwang, MD, (2009), *The Innovator's Prescription: A Disruptive Solution for Health Care*, McGraw Hill Companies, Inc. New York.

109. Dave McComb (2019), 'The Data-Centric Revolution: Restoring Sanity to Entreprise Information Systems', Technics Publications, 2 Lindsley Road, Basking Ridge, NJ 07920, USA

110. Arkady Maydanchik (2007), 'Data Quality Assessment: Data Quality for Practitioners Series', Technics Publications, LLC, Post Office Box 161, Bradley Beach, NJ 07720 USA

111. Arkady Maydanchik (2007) ibid.

112. James Reason (2008), *The Human Contribution: Unsafe Acts, Accidents and Heroic Recoveries*, CRC Press, Taylor Francis Group, Boca Raton, London, New York.

113. Kevin Ashton (2015), *How to Fly a Horse: The Secret History of Invention*, William Heinemann, 20 Vauxhall Bridge Road, London SW1V 2SA.

114. Dave McComb (2019) op cit.

115. Dave McComb (2019), op cit.

116. Werner Vogels (21 June 2018) https://www.allthingsdistributed.com/2018/06/purpose-built-databases-in-aws.html

117. Dave McComb (2018), 'Software Wasteland: How the Application-Centric Mindset is Hobbling our Entreprises', Technics Publications, 2 Lindsley Road, Basking Ridge, NJ 07920, USA

118. Stuart Brand (1995) in Dave McComb (2019), op cit.

119. Dave McComb (2019), op cit.

120. Dave McComb (2019), idid.

121. Werner Vogels (2018), ibid.

122. James C. Scott (1998), 'Seeing Like a State: How Certain Schemes to Improve the Human Condition Have Failed (The Institute for Social Policy St)', Yale University Press

123. Stan Geiger (2018), 'Databases Do Not Build Themselves', http://t.dan.com/databases-do-not-build-themselves/23896

124. In Christensen's language these could be jobs-to-be-done and in J B Fogg's language, if thought through, they could become very specific behaviours to be performed in different contexts.

125. Anita Tucker (2013), 'An Obstacle to Patient Centred Care: Poor Supply Systems', HBR, https://hbr.org/2013/10/an-obstacle-to-patient-centered-care-poor-supply-system.

126. Steven Johnson (2013), 'Recognising the true potential of technology to change behaviour', https://www.theguardian.com/sustainable-business/behavioural-insights/true-potential-technology-change-behaviour.

127. Ian Leslie (2016), The Economist 1843, https://www.1843magazine.com/features/the-scientists-who-make-apps-addictive.

128. See https://www.behaviourmodel.org.

129. Ian Leslie (2016), op cit.

130. B J Fogg (2008), 'Mass Interpersonal Persuasion: An Early View of a New Phenomenon', https://captology.stanford.edu/wp-content/uploads/2014/03/MIP_Fogg_Stanford.pdf.

131. (ibid) B J Fogg (2008).

132. James Reason (2008), The Human Contribution: Unsafe Acts, Accidents and Heroic Recoveries, CRC Press, Taylor Francis Group, Boca Raton, London, New York.

133. Don Norman (2013), The Design of Everyday Things: Revised and Expanded Edition, Basic Books, New York.

134. (ibid) Steven Stack (2017).

135. Dave Gray and Thomas Vander Wal (2014), The Connected Company, O'Reilly Media, 1005 Gravenstein Highway North, Sebastopol, CA 9542.

136. Kevin Ashton (2015), How to Fly a Horse: The Secret History of Invention, William Heinemann, 20 Vauxhall Bridge Road, London SW1V 2SA.

137. B J Fogg (2003), Persuasive Technology: Using Computers to Change What We Think and Do, Morgan Kaufmann Publishers, 340 Pine Street, Sixth Floor, San Francisco, CA 94104-32.

138. B J Fogg (2009), 'A Behavior Model for Persuasive Design', https://www.mebook.se/images/page_file/38/Fogg%20Behavior%20Model.pdf.

139. Gonçalo Veiga (March 21, 2017), 'Intelligence-In-Context: The Rise of Context-Aware Apps', https://www.outsystems.com/blog/intelligence-context-rise-context-aware-apps.html.

140. Manisha Priyadarshini (2018), 'Which sensors do I have in my smartphone? How do they work?', https://fossbytes.com/which-smartphone-sensors-how-work.

141. Anita Tucker (2013), 'An Obstacle to Patient Centred Care: Poor Supply Systems', HBR, https://hbr.org/2013/10/an-obstacle-to-patient-centered-care-poor-supply-systems.

142. Don Norman (2013), The Design of Everyday Things: Revised and Expanded Edition, Basic Books, New York.

143. Australian Government, Australian Institute of Health and Welfare, Australia's Hospitals 2013–14

144. Australia's Health 2018, Australian Government, Australian Institute of Health and Welfare, https://www.aihw.gov.au/reports/australias-health/australias-health-2018/contents/table-of-contents.

145. Manisha Priyadarshini (2018), op cit.

146. Josh Clark (2015), 'Designing for Touch', A Book Apart, New York, https://abookapart.com.

147. Josh Clark (2016), 'Push the possibilities of everyday devices: The Physical Interface', https://bigmedium.com/speaking/the-physical-interface.html.

148. Cindy Stermer, MS, RN-BC, ACNS-BC, Clinical Nurse Specialist (2015), 'Incentivize patients and they will walk', Nursing Affairs, York Hospital, Wellspan Health, York, PA. Telephone: (717) 851-6150., https://www.reliasmedia.com/articles/135692-incentivize-patients-and-they-will-walk.

149. Benedict Evans(2018), 'Ways to think about machine learning', https://www.ben-evans.com/benedictevans/2018/06/22/ways-to-think-about-machine-learning-8nefy.

150. Benedict Evans (2018), 'Ways to think about machine learning', https://www.ben-evans.com/benedictevans/2018/06/22/ways-to-think-about-machine-learning-8nefy.

151. Benedict Evans (2018), op cit.

152. Benedict Evans (2019), 'Finding the point of human leverage', https://www.ben-evans.com/benedictevans/2019/4/8/mechanical-turks.

153. Benedict Evans (2019), op cit.

154. Benedict Evans (2019), 'Does AI make strong tech companies stronger?' https://www.ben-evans.com/benedictevans/2018/12/19/does-ai-make-strong-tech-companies-stronger.

155. Raffaele Iannone, Alfredo Lambiase, Salvatore Miranda, Stefano Riemma, and Debora Sarno (2013), 'Modelling Hospital Materials Management Processes', International Journal of Business Management, Vol 5, 15:2013, https://www.researchgate.net/profile/Debora_Sarno/publication/244484391_Modelling_Hospital_Materials_Management_Processes/links/00b7d51d3f4cadb0f9000000/Modelling-Hospital-Materials-Management-Processes.pdf?origin=publication_detail.

156. Johnathan Bush with Stephen Baker (2014), *Where Does it Hurt: An Entrepreneur's Guide to Fixing Healthcare*, Copyright Athenahealth Inc., Penguin Group, USA

157. Thomas R Krause and John H Hidley (2009), *Taking the Lead in Patient Safety: How Healthcare Leaders Influence Behaviour and Create Culture*, John Wiley & Sons Inc., Hoboken, New Jersey

158. ECRI Institute's 2017 Annual Conference: Workflow, Workarounds, and Overworked Health Systems: Innovations and Challenges for Quality, Safety, and Technology, https://www.youtube.com/playlist?list=PLEvm6gjNpayM15XmCXOCase_gEiUFiSMm.

159. Ontario Hospital Association, 'Optimizing Your Perioperative Supply Chain: A Guide to Improvement Projects'.

160. Session 3: The Role and Influence of Electronic Health Records on Work Burden, ECRI Institute, https://www.youtube.com/watch?v=txt_hmApB-4.

161. Session 4: When Workarounds Are the Norm in Clinical Care, ECRI Institute, https://www.youtube.com/watch?v=sZymhu4_CHE.

162. *Anita Tucker* in Frances Frei, Anne Morriss (2012), *Uncommon Service: How to win by putting customers at the core of your business,* Harvard Business Review Press.

163. Dave Brailsford in James Clear (2018), *Atomic Habits: An Easy and Proven Way to Build Good Habits and Break Bad Ones*, Random House Business Books, The Penguin Random House Group Limited, 20 Vauxhall Bridge Road, London, SW1V 2S.

164. Benedict Evans (2019), 'Finding the point of human leverage', https://www.ben-evans.com/benedictevans/2019/4/8/mechanical-turks.

165. Clayton Christensen, Jerome Grossman and Jason Hwang (2009) ibid.

166. Charles Conn and Robert McLean (2018), *Bulletproof Problem Solving: The One Skill That Changes Everything*, John Wiley & Sons, Inc., Hoboken, New Jersey.

167. Session3: The Role and Influence of Electronic Health Records on Work Burden, ECRI Institute, https://www.youtube.com/watch?v=srqVG5LfFdQ.

168. (ibid) Charles Conn and Robert McLean (2018).

Hidden Hospital Hazard Series

Book 1: *Saving Lives and Improving Margins*

Book 2: *Accurate Procedure Costing and Inventory Management*

Book 3: *Building a Better Business Model*